SUPERFOOD
SMOOTHIE
BOWLS

Delicious, Satisfying, Protein-Packed Blends That Boost Energy and Burn Fat

DANIELLA CHACE

Running Press
PHILADELPHIA · LONDON

D0521429

Published by Running Press,
An Imprint of Perseus Books, LLC.,
A Subsidiary of Hachette Book Group, Inc.

Printed in China

Books published by Running Press are available at special discounts for bulk purchases in the United States by corporations, institutions, and other organizations. For more information, please contact the Special Markets Department at the Perseus Books Group, 2300 Chestnut Street, Suite 200, Philadelphia, PA 19103, or call (800) 810-4145, ext. 5000, or e-mail special.markets@perseusbooks.com.

ISBN 978-0-7624-6106-6
Library of Congress Control Number: 2016934185

E-book ISBN 978-0-7624-6115-8

9 8 7 6 5 4 3 2 1
Digit on the right indicates the number of this printing

Photography by Olivia Brent
Designed by Amanda Richmond
Edited by Kristen Green Wiewora
Typography: Brandon and Sentinel

Running Press Book Publishers
2300 Chestnut Street
Philadelphia, PA 19103-4371

Visit us on the web!
www.offthemenublog.com

FOR TONY CHACE,
MY SWEET DAD,
WHO IS A TRUE
SMOOTHIE BOWL
AFICIONADO.

CONTENTS

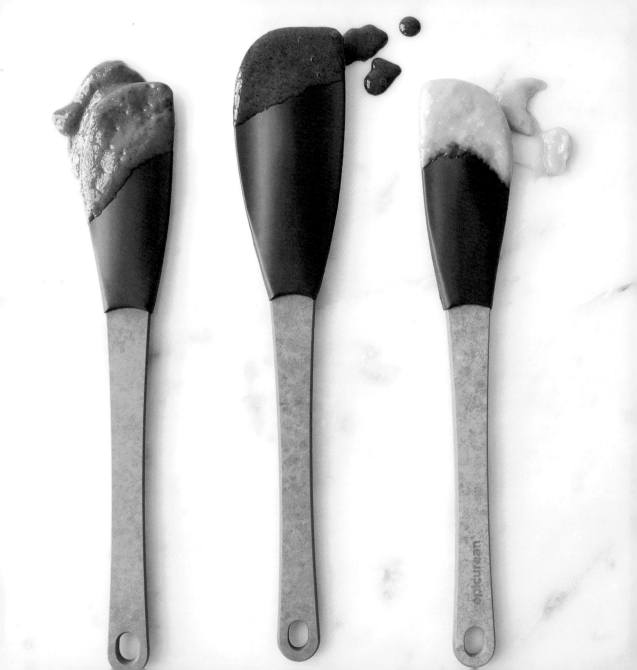

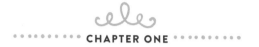

CHAPTER ONE

Introduction

Smoothies are a common element in the diets of the über-healthy. They become a daily ritual for many because they are not only easy to make, but also produce an immediate and noticeable difference in one's health. One reasonable serving size packs in a large quantity of nutrient-rich foods. I'm always impressed by how an entire day's worth of greens purées down to about the size of a tennis ball.

Not only can we ingest a lot of produce in small servings, but we can also choose ingredients that contain high concentrations of all-important phytochemicals, compounds that have the ability to support disease management.

I am a whole foods nutritionist with a passion for functional recipes that are based on findings from empirical scientific research. I've been formulating nutrient-packed smoothies for my clients and readers for decades. Many of my clients report that their daily smoothies boost their energy and improve mood, sleep, skin, memory, and weight loss.

SPOONS, NOT STRAWS

A smoothie bowl is simply a blended smoothie poured into a bowl, complemented with tasty and nutritious toppings. Combining smoothies with whole foods provides nutrients that our bodies can immediately use, as well as fibrous foods that can provide energy for many hours. Enjoying a smoothie bowl will give you longer-lasting energy than you get from a conventional liquid smoothie.

The difference between the way our bodies process whole foods and liquids is significant. Chewing triggers the release of enzymes and acids along the digestive tract, which prepare it for incoming food. Also, whole plant foods contain complex carbohydrates with fiber that metabolizes more slowly, resulting in fewer spikes in blood sugar and insulin.

EVERYONE LOVES A BOWL

A smoothie bowl also has a culinary advantage over a liquid smoothie because eating from a bowl is more like enjoying a meal or dessert than simply drinking a beverage. Kids love smoothie bowls because they have the consistency of ice cream and they can add their favorite toppings, such as berries, fruit, cocoa, or nuts.

THE SUPERFOOD ADVANTAGE

The term *superfoods* is used to identify highly nutritious foods. The foods and food groups that I call superfoods are those that provide physical and mental health benefits. Some of the most exciting superfood research being done today is focused on foods that are widely available. I refer to these studies throughout the recipe chapters as they clearly show us how to use food as medicine.

Ten superfood categories stand out in the current research: berries, citrus, greens, herbs, pomegranate, high-protein sources, spices, stone fruits, tea and coffee, and tropical fruits. This book contains a separate chapter for each superfood.

RECIPES FOR MODERN NEEDS

The recipes found in this book accommodate many dietary restrictions as they are vegan, gluten-free, low in net carbs, and devoid of any kind of common allergenic or synthetic ingredients. Nutrition analysis provides the amount of calories, fats, protein, total carbohydrates, fiber, and the net carbs, which is the amount of sugar producing carbohydrates in the recipe. This is helpful to know as some fiber sources do not produce sugar.

SMOOTHIE BOWL BASICS

A few tips can help you shop for ingredients, set up your pantry, and choose the best tools, so that you can easily create delicious smoothie bowls.

PANTRY

The ingredients used throughout the book are available at most grocery stores, co-ops, and online retailers.

Shop for fresh ingredients once a week, keeping in mind that you will need to use the most delicate (such as greens) quickly, while the heartier items (such as melon or avocado) can last longer. Stock up on nonperishable supplies—spices, dried herbs, protein powders, probiotics, and so on—once a month.

Choose the highest-quality ingredients available in your area, meaning whole rather than packaged, fresh rather than dried, and organic, to ensure minimal exposure to agricultural chemicals. Some produce is more heavily sprayed than others—for example, strawberries—so it's important to look for the certified organic label. Visit the Environmental Working Group (EWG.org) for the Clean Fifteen list (least-sprayed produce) and the Dirty Dozen (the most heavily sprayed).

Opt for unsweetened products, such as cocoa powder, coconut, protein powders, and juices, whenever possible. Also choose ingredients that meet your dietary restrictions, for example, gluten-free granola.

Fresh fruit juices are available in concentrated form in small glass bottles. Concentrates intensify flavor by minimizing the liquid, which also results in a thicker blend. Juice nectars are another great option, as they contain pulp, which adds fiber and flavor to smoothie bowls.

Milks made from seeds and nuts, such as hemp, coconut, and almond, are dairy alternatives that give smoothies a creamy texture. They are found either in the refrigerator section or with the shelf-stable containers that don't require refrigeration until opened. These are usually found in the juice aisle and come plain or flavored. Note that flavored milks are generally higher in sugar.

THE FREEZER

Foods stay fresh for months in the freezer. Freezing seeds and powdered products will help preserve them much longer. Also, chia seeds won't stick to the sides of the blender if used straight from the freezer. Protein and probiotic powders should be frozen to preserve benefits.

STORAGE

Airtight food storage containers are a good investment because they keep foods from oxidizing, which means they will stay fresh longer. Dry foods can be safely stored in plastic, though glass is preferable for all food storage. Containers with airtight seals can be used for dry products, such as nuts, chia seeds, and protein powder.

My countertop containers store my tea, nuts, seeds, and everyday spices. I use smaller glass jars for spices that I only use occasionally and place them in the cupboard, out of the light, where they will last longer.

Glass refrigerator and freezer containers are your best option for storing wet or acidic foods, both of which have the potential to leach phthalates from plastics. Look for tempered glass, such as Duralex, which won't break in the freezer.

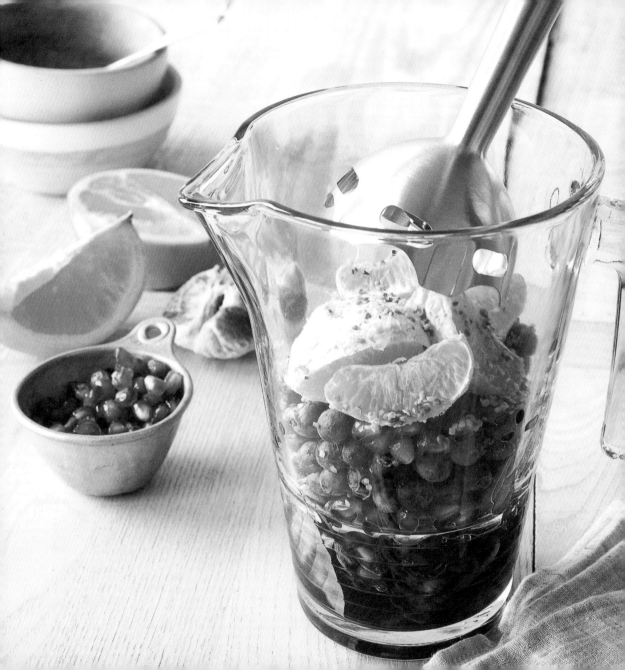

MANDOLINE

SPICE GRATER

GRATER

ZESTER

MICROPLANE

KITCHEN TOOLS

All that's really needed to make smoothie bowls is a blender, a cutting board, and a knife for prepping produce. Well-made tools, however, make the process safer and easier. I also recommend the following helpful accessories.

BLENDERS

Blenders vary in their power levels. Lower-powered blenders work better with soft ingredients, such as fresh fruits. They may require extra liquid to ease strain on the motor. Higher-powered blenders have a much easier time blending frozen fruits and whole nuts, even without extra liquids. When choosing a blender, look for glass or stainless-steel pitchers, which are free of the phthalates that are inherent in plastic pitchers. If your blender has a plastic pitcher, there is still minimal health risk as long as the plastic doesn't get hot.

If you want to be able to blend frozen foods easily, get a high-powered blender.

If you prefer fresh produce in your smoothies, a low-powered blender will be sufficient. Immersion or handheld blenders can also be used to make smoothies right in a bowl, provided the bowl is unbreakable and deep enough that the blend doesn't splatter. Immersion blenders are lightweight and often come with attachments for making not only smoothies, but also whipped cream and creamed soup. Always make sure the immersion blender is unplugged before cleaning or handling anywhere near the blade.

KNIVES & SLICERS

A high-quality knife is an essential tool to have in the kitchen, as prepping fresh produce is easier with a sharp, sturdy knife.

I use a 6-inch blade for almost all of my chopping. Never run your knives through the dishwasher, as this can dull the blades and damage the handles. Always rinse, dry, and put them away after each use to avoid dropping or damaging the blades.

Quality knives, such as Shun, Wüsthof,

and Messermeister, are made of stainless steel, so they require less sharpening than softer materials.

A Microplane can be used to dust a soft powdering of nutritious citrus peel over a bowl, and a zester allows you to grate bright shavings of peel over the top of your bowls. A stainless-steel grater will give you larger pieces of peel, while a mandoline slicer makes wide, thin slices. Use a spice grater to grate hard spices, such as nutmeg, to provide more flavor and fragrance than pre-ground spices.

CUTTING BOARDS

Choose a large cutting board for preparing produce so food doesn't spill off the edges as you work. Avoid plastic boards, as they can release toxic phthalates into food, and wooden boards, which develop deep grooves where bacteria can grow. Pressed paper boards are nontoxic and preserve knife edges better than harder boards. I use Epicurean cutting boards as they last for years even with daily washing.

MEASURING TOOLS

Look for glass or stainless-steel measuring cups and spoons, avoiding those that are chrome-plated, plastic, or aluminum, all of which can degrade or release toxins into foods over time.

BOWLS

Keep a variety of bowls on hand: larger bowls for "meal" smoothies and smaller ones for appetizers and desserts. Shatterproof glass, such as Duralex brand, are strong enough to use with an immersion blender and come in many sizes.

ICE CUBE TRAYS

I use nontoxic silicone ice cube trays, such as Lékué brand, to freeze leftover smoothies, juices, nut milks, and even steamed greens for later use.

SPATULAS

You'll want spatulas handy to get every last drop of smoothie from your blender. Opt for silicone over plastic, as it is nontoxic.

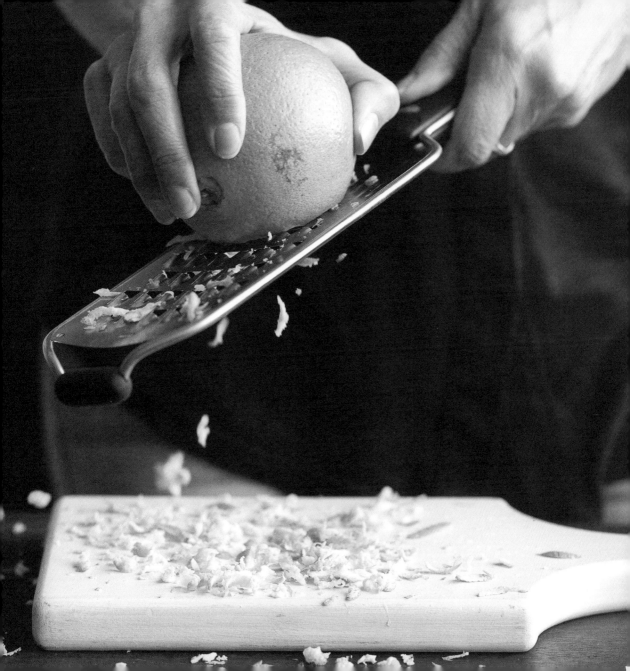

ASSEMBLING A SMOOTHIE BOWL

There are three basic steps to assembling a smoothie bowl: prepping the ingredients, blending the smoothie ingredients, and sprinkling the blended smoothie with your desired toppings. Here are some tips to help you get the most nutrition from your ingredients and a few tricks of the trade that I have learned along the way.

PREPPING

Prepare your produce by washing, removing pits, and chopping as necessary.

Nutrients are concentrated in various parts of plants: in their fruit's peel, leaves, roots, and seeds. The peel of fruits often contains a higher concentration of medicinally active compounds than the fruit. Citrus peels and banana peels are packed with flavonoids and melatonin, respectively. Adding more of the superdense parts of plants to smoothies increases the nutritional value considerably.

Citrus and banana peels are included in several recipes as a suggestion for those who are adventurous in the kitchen. Banana peel adds herbal-like flavor, and citrus peel packs a wallop of fragrance to smoothies. Be sure that any peel used is organic, wash it well, and chop it unless using a high-powered blender. One tablespoon of peel per serving is the ideal amount to add, as this boosts nutrition and adds flavor and fragrance without overloading the recipe with too much fiber or bitter compounds.

I mentioned packaged nut milks earlier, but I highly recommend you try making your own. The flavor of homemade milks is much fresher than store-bought products. All you need are nuts, water, and a mesh nut-milk bag. Blend one part nuts with four parts water, pour into the bag, then squeeze the nut milk out into a container with a lid, and refrigerate. This will keep, refrigerated, for about four days.

Likewise, fruit and vegetable juices can be made at home with a juicer; this provides a higher nutrient content and

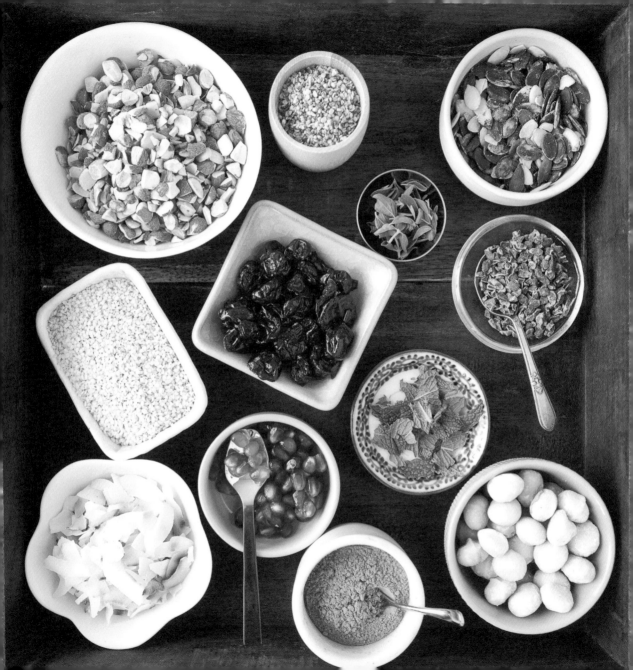

fresher flavor than store-bought juices.

You can freeze tea, juices, and nut milks in silicone ice cube trays for later use.

Spritz fresh herbs with water, wrap in a clean cloth, and place in the refrigerator to maintain freshness. Greens can be lightly steamed first to ease blending and to improve the bioavailability of their nutrients.

For best results, soak nuts overnight in water before blending.

Grind whole spices, using a spice mill or coffee grinder.

Before blending, remove pits and stems from fruit. Store-bought frozen stone fruit are already pitted, making them a convenient ingredient for smoothies.

Large pits must be removed and the skin discarded from such fruits as mango and avocado. The skin and flesh of soft fruits, such as bananas and star fruit, can be blended whole. The skin from melon and dragon fruit should be peeled before blending the flesh. Most seeds can be directly added to any blend.

BLENDING

When you have all your ingredients ready, begin by adding the liquids to the blender. Doing so will reduce pressure on low-powered motors. Next, add any soft ingredients, such as fresh fruits and vegetables, followed by tougher, frozen, or drier ingredients, such as pomegranate arils (a.k.a. seeds), frozen berries, and nuts.

Frozen ingredients may bog down the blender motor. If this happens, add a little water and let the ingredients thaw for a few minutes before continuing. Even high-powered blenders can get stuck when a majority of the ingredients are frozen. Frozen fruit can be replaced with fresh in any of the recipes; however, frozen fruit will yield a thicker, frostier blend.

The difference between making a smoothie for a bowl rather than a glass is the consistency. Bowl smoothies need to have a thick blend, similar to yogurt, rather than being liquefied, like a beverage. There are several ways to thicken a smoothie for a bowl. Creamy ingredients, such as nut butters, hulled hemp seeds, and avocado, add body to a blend. Protein powders and chia seeds soak up extra liquid, thickening it. Frozen fruit, such as bananas, work very well in creating a soft, ice cream–like texture. Also, simply reducing the amount of liquid used can thicken many smoothie recipes.

Once you have blended the ingredients, pour the smoothie into bowls, and add the toppings.

TOPPING

Chop or slice your choice of toppings, assemble atop the smoothie, and serve your bowls ready to eat. Or, if you're serving the dishes to others, set out the toppings and let them design their bowls according to their tastes and needs.

Topping options include crunchy bits, such as sliced almonds, pumpkin seeds, coconut flakes, and cocoa nibs; fresh fruits, such as banana, pomegranate arils, and juicy mango; fragrant herbs and spices, including mint, cinnamon, basil, and vanilla. You can top the whole thing off with your favorite powder, for example, cocoa or matcha (ground green tea leaves). All add scent, flavor, and texture to your blend.

It's important to eat your bowls right after making them. Blending cuts the plants' fibers, which causes the nutrients to oxidize from exposure to oxygen, reducing their potency—so eat up!

PERSONALIZE YOUR BOWL

You can create personalized recipes by combining foods that contain nutrients to meet your own—or your loved ones'—tastes and health goals. You can add foods to your smoothie bowls that contain the specific biochemicals that address your dietary needs. For example, those with anemia can throw in spinach for its iron content; those with dry skin might add in avocado and probiotic powder. Consult the section entitled "Personalized

Therapeutic Smoothie Bowls" (page 183) for a full list of ingredients and the conditions they support. And be sure to read the recipe sidebars for more about the nutrients provided by particular ingredients.

A BOWL FOR EVERY OCCASION

Savory smoothie bowls can be served as small, healthy appetizers. The sorbet and herb bowls make excellent palate cleansers. Dessert bowls work equally well for children or dinner party guests. You can treat yourself to dessert without guilt, while quelling cravings for more sugar-laden treats. Smoothie bowls also make a perfect after-school snack. I love the coffee and tea bowls on warm summer days, when cold food is more appealing than hot drinks.

Indulge frequently in smoothie bowls as they are not only guilt-free pleasures, but are also sufficiently nourishing that they can be considered an essential part of health protection and disease management.

A daily smoothie bowl is a simple habit to develop and maintain. While you are enjoying your delicious bowl of fresh fruits, nuts, greens, herbs, and spices, rest assured that you are also providing your body with a whole pharmacy of healthful nutrients. A personalized smoothie bowl nourishes, detoxifies, calms the mind, fights disease, supports an active lifestyle, and supplies you with the energy and vigor to face the challenges of the modern world.

And smoothie bowls are such fun to make! Time to get out your bowls and start blending!

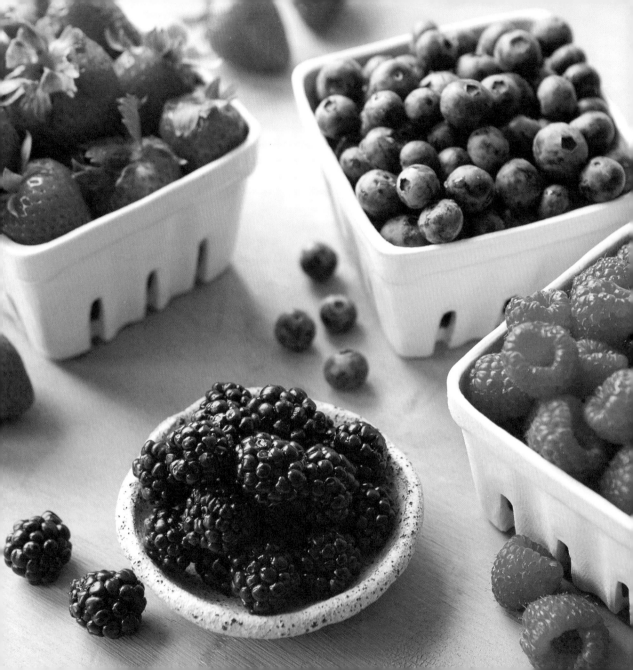

CHAPTER

2

BERRY BOWL RECIPES

Blueberry Cream

This classic combination is rich in flavor and nutrients. Coconut milk yogurt adds a delicious creaminess as well as probiotics to aid in digestion.

Serves 2

SMOOTHIE
1 banana, peeled
1 cup blueberries
$^1/_2$ cup coconut milk yogurt
$^1/_4$ cup hulled hemp seeds
1 teaspoon ground cinnamon

Combine all the ingredients in a blender and blend until smooth.

TOPPINGS
$^1/_4$ cup peeled, sliced banana
$^1/_4$ cup sliced strawberries
2 tablespoons hulled hemp seeds
2 tablespoons sliced almonds

Pour the smoothie into two small bowls, sprinkle each with half of the toppings, and serve.

NUTRITION FACTS (GRAMS PER SERVING)
Calories 350, Fat 20, Protein 14, Carbs 33, Fiber 8, NetCarbs 25

Probiotics, such as those found in cultured foods, reduce inflammation in the gastro-intestinal tract and significantly lower the risk for development of colon cancer as well as support proper hydration.

Superfood Granola Bowl

This bowl is a sweet blend with warming cinnamon. Peaches and blueberries deliver powerful antioxidants to help fight free radicals.

Serves 2

SMOOTHIE

1 cup sliced peach

1 cup blueberries

1/2 cup coconut milk yogurt

1/4 cup chia seeds

1 tablespoon ground cinnamon

Combine all the ingredients in a blender and blend until smooth.

TOPPINGS

1/2 cup blueberries

2 tablespoons granola

2 tablespoons toasted pumpkin seeds

2 tablespoons hulled hemp seeds

Pour the smoothie into two small bowls and sprinkle each with half of the toppings and serve.

NUTRITION FACTS (GRAMS PER SERVING)
Calories 310, Fat 17, Protein 11, Carbs 33, Fiber 12, NetCarbs 21

Antioxidants counteract the negative impact of reactive molecules known as free radicals. Oxidative stress is a primary cause of neurodegenerative disorders, such as dementia and Alzheimer's disease. Daily intake of antioxidant-rich foods reduces oxidation and protects the brain from the damage that leads to memory loss.

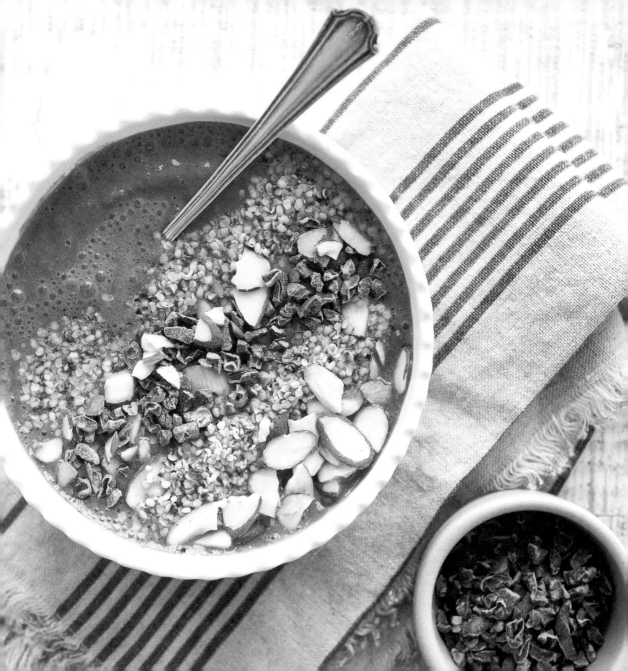

Chocolate-Covered Cherries

A nutrient-dense treat, this bowl blends
antioxidant-rich cherries and cocoa into delicious perfection.

Serves 2

SMOOTHIE

2 cups pitted dark sweet cherries

$1/2$ cup almond milk

$1/4$ cup hulled hemp seeds

1 tablespoon unsweetened cocoa powder

Combine all the ingredients in a blender and blend until smooth.

TOPPINGS

2 tablespoons sliced almonds

2 tablespoons hulled hemp seeds

2 teaspoons cocoa nibs

Pour the smoothie into two small bowls and sprinkle each with half of the toppings and serve.

NUTRITION FACTS (GRAMS PER SERVING)
Calories 250, Fat 19, Protein 12, Carbs 12, Fiber 4, NetCarbs 18

Seventy percent of the population has hypertension by age seventy and this is accompanied by oxidative stress. Dietary intake of foods rich in vitamin C, vitamin E, carotenoids, polyphenols, and trace elements are known to have high antioxidant potency that assist in minimizing harmful effects of free radicals, providing therapeutic and preventive benefits.

Summer Picnic

This bowl has the perfect combination of almond and berry flavors and its chia seeds are a dense source of anti-inflammatory oils.

Serves 2

SMOOTHIE

1/4 lemon, chopped with peel (seeds removed)

1 cup strawberry halves

1 cup blueberries

1/4 cup almond milk

1/4 cup chia seeds

2 tablespoons almond butter

Combine all the ingredients in a blender and blend until smooth.

TOPPINGS

1/2 cup sliced strawberries

2 tablespoons sliced almonds

2 tablespoons hulled hemp seeds

Pour the smoothie into two small bowls and sprinkle each with half of the toppings and serve.

NUTRITION FACTS (GRAMS PER SERVING)
Calories 430, Fat 23 , Protein 17, Carbs 38, Fiber 20, NetCarbs 18

Chia seeds provide 3 grams of protein, 6 grams of fiber, and 3 grams of omega oils in just 1 tablespoon. Their omega-3 fatty acids decrease the production of inflammatory cytokines and eicosanoids, which are implicated in chronic inflammatory autoimmune diseases, such as Crohn's disease, ankylosing spondylitis, and rheumatoid arthritis. Daily intake of omega-3s reduces the progression of these diseases as well as associated pain.

Cherry Pecan Cream

Creamy and light, this bowl delivers serious probiotic benefits
to support improved mood, better sleep, and increased immunity.

Serves 2

SMOOTHIE

1 banana, peeled

1 cup pitted dark sweet cherries

$1/2$ cup coconut milk yogurt

$1/4$ cup chia seeds

1 teaspoon probiotic powder

Combine all the ingredients in a blender and blend until smooth.

TOPPINGS

$1/2$ cup peeled, sliced banana

2 tablespoons unsweetened flaked coconut

2 tablespoons chopped pecans

Pour the smoothie into two small bowls and sprinkle each with half of the toppings and serve.

NUTRITION FACTS (GRAMS PER SERVING)
Calories 260, Fat 15, Protein 8, Carbs 32, Fiber 15, NetCarbs 17

Coconut milk yogurt contains probiotic organisms, such as those found in probiotic supplements and yogurt. These healthful organisms support sleep, relaxation, and immunity and reduce inflammation throughout the body. They also influence memory, mood, and cognition and are clinically and therapeutically relevant to a range of disorders, including chronic fatigue syndrome, fibromyalgia, restless leg syndrome, and alcoholism.

Berry Blood Orange Bowl

Tart and citrusy, this bowl contains berry compounds
that help protect and heal the heart from cardiovascular disease.

Serves 2

SMOOTHIE

1 cup blood orange segments
1 cup raspberries
$1/2$ cup blackberries
$1/4$ cup protein powder
3 tablespoons black cherry
juice concentrate

Combine all the ingredients in
a blender and blend until smooth.

TOPPINGS

$1/2$ cup raspberries
1 tablespoon orange zest
Sprigs of fresh mint leaves

Pour the smoothie into two small
bowls and sprinkle each with half
of the toppings and serve.

NUTRITION FACTS (GRAMS PER SERVING)
Calories 159, Fat 0, Protein 14, Carbs 24, Fiber 10, NetCarbs 14

Berries, such as strawberries, raspberries, blackberries, blueberries, and cranberries,
are unrivaled sources of bioactive compounds, such as phenolic acids, anthocyanins,
and flavonols, which prevent inflammatory disorders and cardiovascular diseases, and
lower the risk of various cancers.

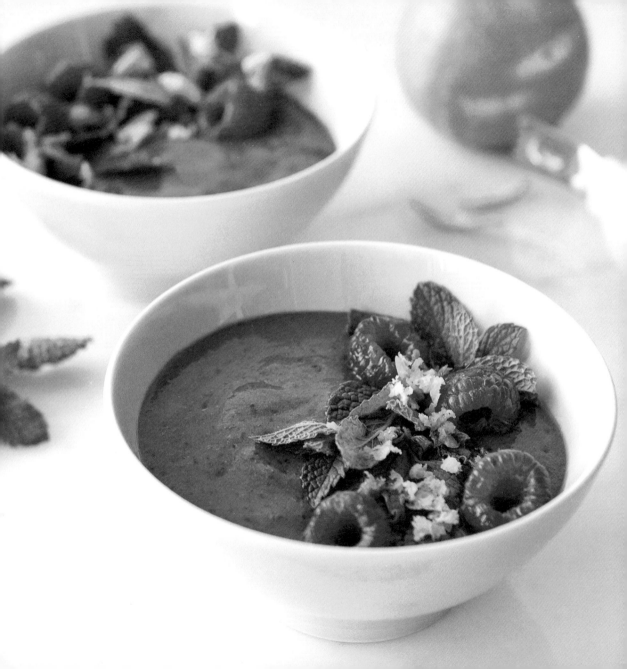

Lemon Berry Sorbet

This blend of rich berry with tart citrus
lemon flavor tastes like an Italian sorbet.

Serves 2

SMOOTHIE

¹/4 lemon, chopped with peel
(seeds removed)
1 cup fresh spinach leaves
1 cup blueberries
1 cup strawberry halves
¹/4 cup chia seeds
3 tablespoons black cherry
juice concentrate

Combine all the ingredients in
a blender and blend until smooth.

TOPPINGS

¹/2 cup raspberries
2 tablespoons toasted sliced almonds
2 tablespoons hulled hemp seeds

Pour the smoothie into two small
bowls and sprinkle each with half
of the toppings and serve.

NUTRITION FACTS (GRAMS PER SERVING)
Calories 340, Fat 19, Protein 13, Carbs 39, Fiber 18, NetCarbs 21

This bowl has a synergistic blend of iron-rich spinach and vitamin C—rich fruits that
help reverse anemia and support those with hypothyroid function.

Tangerine Burst

This bowl is bright and citrusy with sweet, crunchy toppings.
A delicious combination of foods that contain compounds that support vision.

Serves 2

SMOOTHIE

2 cups tangerine segments

1 cup strawberry halves

1/2 cup fresh spinach leaves

1/2 cup carrot juice

1/4 cup hulled hemp seeds

Combine all the ingredients in a blender and blend until smooth.

TOPPINGS

1/2 cup sliced strawberries

1/2 cup shredded carrots

2 tablespoons toasted hulled hemp seeds

Pour the smoothie into two small bowls and sprinkle each with half of the toppings and serve.

NUTRITION FACTS (GRAMS PER SERVING)
Calories 280, Fat 14, Protein 12, Carbs 30, Fiber 7, NetCarbs 23

Carrot juice is an excellent source of the carotenoid nutrients lutein and zeaxanthin, which have a protective effect against cataracts and retinopathy.

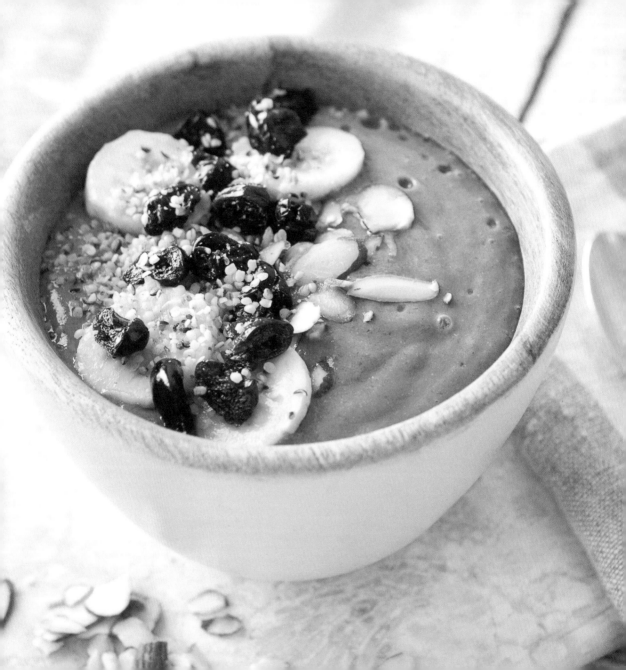

Midsummer Sorbet

This smoothie bowl has rich berry flavor reminiscent
of an Italian sorbet and powerful anti-inflammatory benefits.

Serves 2

SMOOTHIE

1 banana, peeled

1 cup raspberries

1 cup pitted dark sweet cherries

$1/4$ cup hulled hemp seeds

3 tablespoons black cherry
juice concentrate

Combine all the ingredients in
a blender and blend until smooth.

TOPPINGS

$1/2$ cup peeled, sliced banana

2 tablespoons sliced almonds

2 tablespoons hulled hemp seeds

2 tablespoons chopped dried cherries

Pour the smoothie into two small
bowls and sprinkle each with half
of the toppings and serve.

NUTRITION FACTS (GRAMS PER SERVING)
Calories 350, Fat 17, Protein 13, Carbs 39, Fiber 10, NetCarbs 29

Ellagic acid is an antioxidant polyphenol derived from berries and nuts that is effective
at reducing inflammation.

Berry Mint Greens

Sweet strawberries and kale add bright color and fresh garden flavor to this nutrient-dense bowl that contains nutrients that modify blood fats and sugar.

Serves 2

SMOOTHIE

2 fresh kale leaves, ribs removed
1 cup strawberry halves
$1/2$ cup raspberries
$1/2$ cup hemp milk
$1/4$ cup hulled hemp seeds

Combine all the ingredients in a blender and blend until smooth.

TOPPINGS

$1/2$ cup sliced strawberries
2 tablespoons hulled hemp seeds
Sprigs of fresh mint leaves

Pour the smoothie into two small bowls and sprinkle each with half of the toppings and serve.

NUTRITION FACTS (GRAMS PER SERVING)
Calories 220, Fat 14, Protein 11, Carbs 15, Fiber 6, NetCarbs 9

Berries provide vitamins C and E, selenium, calcium, and soluble and insoluble fiber, and have only around 40 calories in a half cup. Strawberries also deliver beta-glucans, which have been found to reduce cholesterol, increase weight loss, improve insulin sensitivity, and control blood sugar.

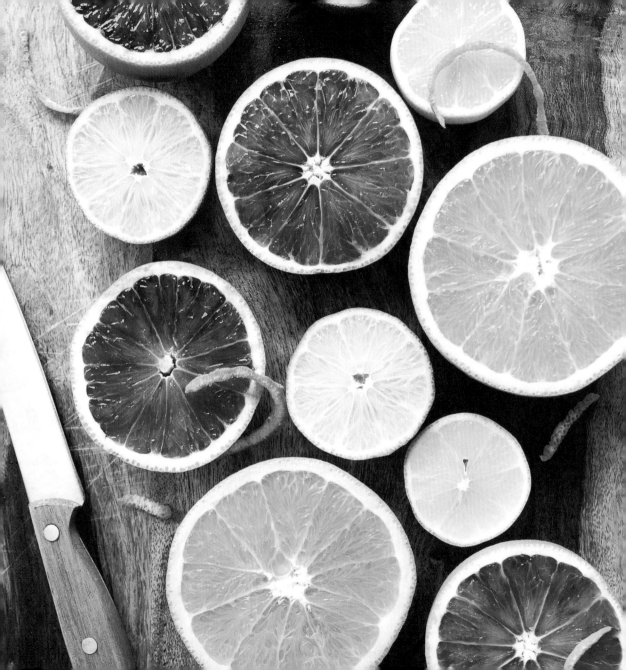

3

CITRUS
BOWL
RECIPES

Orange Chocolate Mousse

This tart, creamy blend contains bioactive molecules from cocoa, which have been shown to help lower the risk of heart disease.

Serves 2

SMOOTHIE

1 banana, peeled
1 cup orange segments
$^1/_2$ cup coconut milk yogurt
$^1/_4$ cup protein powder
$^1/_4$ cup hulled hemp seeds
2 tablespoons unsweetened cocoa powder

Combine all the ingredients in a blender and blend until smooth.

TOPPINGS

2 tablespoons hulled hemp seeds
2 teaspoons cocoa nibs
Sprigs of fresh mint leaves

Pour the smoothie into two small bowls and sprinkle each with half of the toppings and serve.

NUTRITION FACTS (GRAMS PER SERVING)
Calories 270, Fat 11, Protein 20, Carbs 30, Fiber 10, NetCarbs 20

Cardiovascular disease is the most common cause of death in the Western world. Polyphenols, prevalently contained in foods, such as cocoa, fruits, and green tea, are associated with lowered cardiovascular risk factors including reduction of oxidative stress, platelet aggregation, blood pressure, and cholesterol.

Ginger Berry Sorbet

A mouthwatering combination of citrus, berries, and ginger, this blend contains powerful food compounds that provide protection for blood sugar imbalances.

Serves 2

SMOOTHIE

1 cup orange segments

1 (1-inch) piece ginger root, peeled and minced

1 cup blueberries

$1/4$ cup chia seeds

3 tablespoons black cherry juice concentrate

Combine all the ingredients in a blender and blend until smooth.

TOPPINGS

$1/2$ cup tangerine segments

2 tablespoons chopped candied ginger

Sprigs of fresh mint leaves

Pour the smoothie into two small bowls and sprinkle each with half of the toppings and serve.

NUTRITION FACTS (GRAMS PER SERVING)
Calories 250, Fat 11, Protein 8, Carbs 38, Fiber 16, NetCarbs 22

Ginger contains the bioactive compounds shogaol and gingerol, which have been found to protect against diabetes-related complications, such as neurological damage, for those with type 1 or type 2 diabetes.

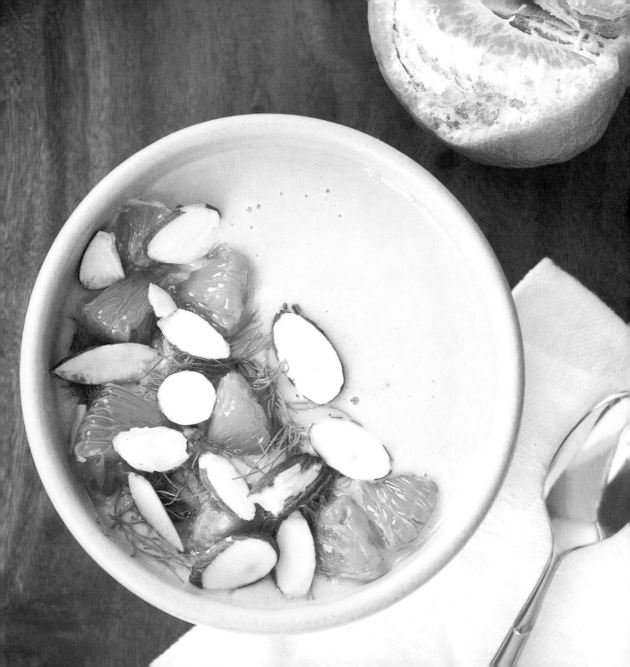

Licorice Citrus

Sweet tangerine and fennel blend together in this bright bowl loaded with protective, anti-inflammatory properties from the peel of citrus fruits.

Serves 2

SMOOTHIE

2 cups mandarin orange segments

$1/2$ banana, peeled

2 tablespoons grated mandarin orange zest

$1/2$ cup chopped fennel bulb

$1/4$ cup tangerine juice

$1/4$ cup hulled hemp seeds

Combine all the ingredients in a blender and blend until smooth.

TOPPINGS

2 tablespoons tangerine segments

2 tablespoons toasted sliced almond

Sprigs of fresh fennel greens

Pour the smoothie into two small bowls and sprinkle each with half of the toppings and serve.

NUTRITION FACTS (GRAMS PER SERVING)
Calories 167, Fat 6, Protein 6, Carbs 23, Fiber 6, NetCarbs 17

Tangeretin, a flavonoid in citrus fruits and their peels, has been proven to play an important role in anti-inflammatory responses and provides neuroprotective effects.

Pomelo Punch

This tart, citrus-packed bowl provides antimicrobial nutrients
and immune-boosting compounds. Top it with
delicious and crunchy pomegranate arils and pumpkin seeds.

Serves 2

SMOOTHIE	TOPPINGS
1 cup tangerine segments	$1/2$ cup orange segments
1 cup pomelo segments	2 tablespoons pomegranate arils
1 cup blueberries	2 tablespoons pumpkin seeds
$1/4$ cup pomegranate juice	
$1/4$ cup chia seeds	

Combine all the ingredients in a blender and blend until smooth.

Pour the smoothie into two small bowls and sprinkle each with half of the toppings and serve.

NUTRITION FACTS (GRAMS PER SERVING)
Calories 340, Fat 16, Protein 11, Carbs 45, Fiber 18, NetCarbs 27

The juice, pulp, and peel from tangerines, grapes, lemon, and lime contain alkaloids, flavonoids, steroids, terpenoids, saponins, and glycosides that provide antimicrobial activities against bacteria and fungus.

Good Morning Grapefruit

This tart grapefruit blend wakes up the digestive tract and gives the metabolism a jump start on the day.

Serves 2

SMOOTHIE

2 cups grapefruit segments
1 cup blueberries
$1/2$ cup currant juice
$1/4$ cup chia seeds

Combine all the ingredients in a blender and blend until smooth.

TOPPINGS

$1/2$ cup tangerine segments
2 tablespoons sliced almonds
2 tablespoons unsweetened flaked coconut

Pour the smoothie into two small bowls and sprinkle each with half of the toppings and serve.

NUTRITION FACTS (GRAMS PER SERVING)
Calories 300, Fat 14, Protein 9, Carbs 41, Fiber 16, NetCarbs 25

Grapefruit contains bioactive flavonoids, such as naringin and isonaringin, which support weight loss and reduce hyperinsulinemia via their outstanding antioxidant activity.

Blood Orange Blast

Stimulating ginger and bright parsley blend perfectly
with blood oranges in this refreshing blend. The fiber-rich toppings
help reduce weight gain and lower blood pressure.

Serves 2

SMOOTHIE

2 cups blood orange segments

1 (1-inch) piece ginger root,
peeled and minced

1 cup raspberries

1/2 cup fresh flat-leaf parsley leaves

1/4 cup chia seeds

3 tablespoons currant juice

Combine all the ingredients in
a blender and blend until smooth.

TOPPINGS

2 tablespoons sliced almonds

2 tablespoons unsweetened
flaked coconut

Sprigs of fresh flat-leaf
parsley leaves

Pour the smoothie into two small
bowls and sprinkle each with half
of the toppings and serve.

NUTRITION FACTS (GRAMS PER SERVING)
Calories 226, Fat 9, Protein 9, Carbs 35, Fiber 19, NetCarbs 16

Berries, nuts, and coconut are all sources of fiber that decrease the risk of obesity, hyper-cholesterolemia, and high blood pressure.

Mandarin Basil Velvet

A velvety combination that is both sweet and herbal, this bowl contains bioactives that provide protection against many age-related diseases.

Serves 2

SMOOTHIE
2 cups mandarin orange segments
1 cup red grapes
1 cup fresh basil leaves
$1/4$ cup chia seeds
3 tablespoons currant juice

Combine all the ingredients in a blender and blend until smooth.

TOPPINGS
$1/2$ cup peeled, sliced banana
$1/2$ cup pitted, peeled, and chopped mango
2 tablespoons unsweetened flaked coconut

Pour the smoothie into two small bowls and sprinkle each with half of the toppings and serve.

NUTRITION FACTS (GRAMS PER SERVING)
Calories 280, Fat 11, Protein 8, Carbs 45, Fiber 16, NetCarbs 29

Red grapes provide resveratrol, which is a well-studied phytophenol antioxidant with beneficial effects in the prevention of cardiovascular diseases, cancer, inflammation, and eye diseases, such as age-related macular degeneration. Resveratrol is the purple pigment found in the skin and seeds of grapes, plums, berries, pomegranates, walnuts, pistachios, and cocoa.

Vanilla Pumpkin Cream

A satisfying bowl with a synergistic combination of nutrients to protect
the skin and reduce wrinkles, this blend has complex flavors and fragrance.
Topped with fresh strawberries and pumpkin seeds to enhance the benefits.

Serves 2

SMOOTHIE

2 bananas, peeled

$^1/_4$ lime, chopped with peel
(seeds removed)

$^1/_2$ cup carrot juice

$^1/_4$ hulled hemp seeds

$^1/_4$ cup pumpkin seeds

2 teaspoons pure vanilla extract

Combine all the ingredients in
a blender and blend until smooth.

TOPPINGS

$^1/_2$ cup sliced strawberries

2 tablespoons pumpkin seeds

2 tablespoons toasted flaked coconut

Pour the smoothie into two small
bowls and sprinkle each with half
of the toppings and serve.

NUTRITION FACTS (GRAMS PER SERVING)
Calories 380, Fat 22, Protein 16, Carbs 39, Fiber 6, NetCarbs 33

Researchers have discovered that even small doses of vitamin C, zinc, and carotenoids
make a marked improvement in skin health and a visible reduction of wrinkles after
just a few weeks of daily intake. This blend contains all three: strawberries (vitamin C),
pumpkin seeds (zinc), and carrot juice (carotenoids).

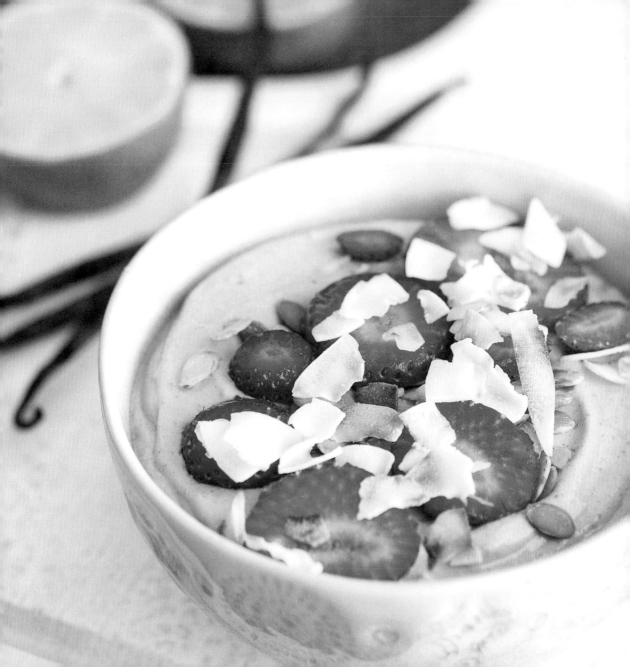

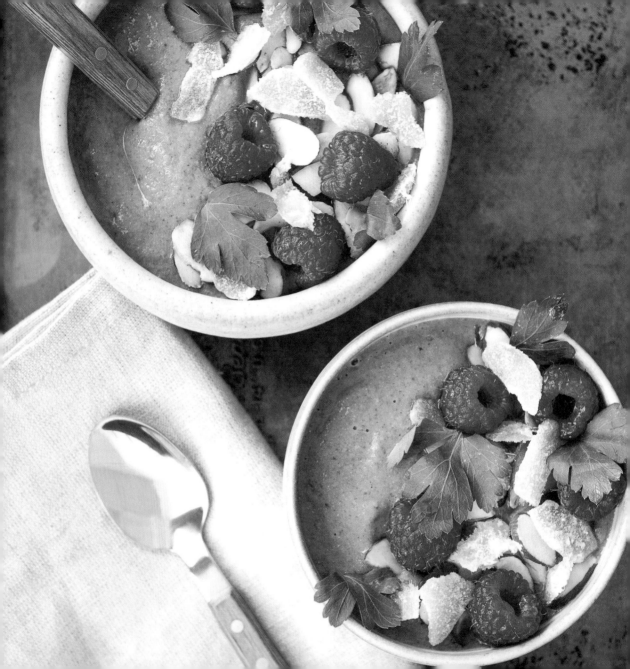

Fall Sunshine

This mood-lifting bowl is rich in the flavors of fall,
such as spiced cider, leafy greens, and winter oranges.

Serves 2

SMOOTHIE

2 cups orange segments

2 fresh kale leaves, ribs removed

1 cup sliced apple

1 (1-inch) piece turmeric root, peeled and minced

1/4 cup chia seeds

3 tablespoons unfiltered apple juice

Pinch of freshly ground black pepper

Combine all the ingredients in a blender and blend until smooth.

TOPPINGS

1/2 cup raspberries

2 tablespoons sliced almonds

2 tablespoons candied ginger

Sprigs of fresh flat-leaf parsley leaves

Pour the smoothie into two small bowls and sprinkle each with half of the toppings and serve.

NUTRITION FACTS (GRAMS PER SERVING)
Calories 280, Fat 14, Protein 9, Carbs 40, Fiber 20, NetCarbs 20

Major depression is a common, recurrent, and chronic disease that negatively affects quality of life. Studies have demonstrated that curcumin, the yellow-pigmented substance found in turmeric, possesses antidepressant properties. Black pepper contains the bioactive piperine, which enhances the absorption of curcumin, making it even more effective.

Grapefruit Kiwi Boost

A grapefruit lover's delight, this balanced bowl is a bioactive
mix of plant compounds that help reduce harmful bacteria in the body.

Serves 2

SMOOTHIE	TOPPINGS
3 kiwi, peeled	1/2 cup peeled, sliced banana
1 banana, peeled	2 tablespoons hulled hemp seeds
1/4 grapefruit with peel (seeds removed)	1 teaspoon fresh thyme leaves
1/4 cup hemp milk	
1/4 cup hulled hemp seeds	

Combine all the ingredients in a blender and blend until smooth.

Pour the smoothie into two small bowls and sprinkle each with half of the toppings and serve.

NUTRITION FACTS (GRAMS PER SERVING)
Calories 283, Fat 10, Protein 10, Carbs 38, Fiber 8, NetCarbs 30

Both dried and fresh thyme leaves contain bioactive compounds that reduce fungal and bacterial growth.

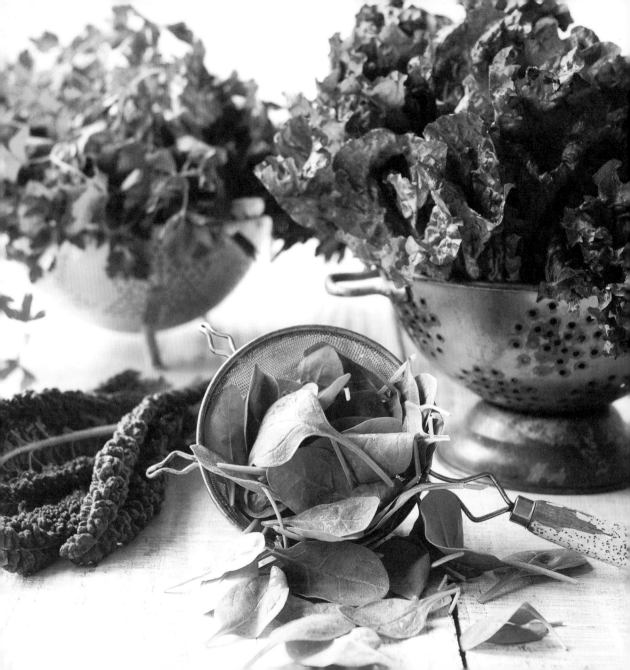

GREEN BOWL RECIPES

Super Strawberry Citrus

This bowl has luscious strawberry and citrus
flavor and an energizing nutrient combination.

Serves 2

SMOOTHIE

1 tangerine

2 cups strawberry halves

$1/2$ cup fresh spinach leaves

$1/4$ cup chia seeds

3 tablespoons cherry juice concentrate

Combine all the ingredients in
a blender and blend until smooth.

TOPPINGS

$1/2$ cup sliced strawberries

$1/2$ cup tangerine segments

2 tablespoons hulled hemp seeds

Pour the smoothie into two small
bowls and sprinkle each with half
of the toppings and serve.

NUTRITION FACTS (GRAMS PER SERVING)
Calories 340, Fat 19, Protein 15, Carbs 36, Fiber 18, Net Carbs 18

CULINARY TIP: The color will be brighter with fresh strawberries than with frozen.

Even in industrialized countries, iron-deficiency anemia is common. Anemia causes
such symptoms as foggy memory, cold hands and feet, pale skin, and fatigue. Daily intake
of iron-rich foods, such as spinach, combined with foods containing vitamin C, such as
citrus and strawberries, improve the absorption of iron and help prevent anemia.

Almond Blueberry Calmer

Nutty and sweet, this bowl provides
stress-reducing magnesium from almonds and fresh spinach.

Serves 2

SMOOTHIE

$^1/_2$ banana, peeled

1 cup blueberries

$^1/_2$ cup fresh spinach leaves

$^1/_4$ cup almond milk

$^1/_4$ cup toasted hulled hemp seeds

Combine all the ingredients in
a blender and blend until smooth.

TOPPINGS

$^1/_4$ cup blueberries

2 tablespoons sliced almonds

2 tablespoons toasted hulled
hemp seeds

Pour the smoothie into two small
bowls and sprinkle each with half
of the toppings and serve.

NUTRITION FACTS (GRAMS PER SERVING)
Calories 200, Fat 10, Protein 8, Carbs 23, Fiber 5, NetCarbs 18

Magnesium plays an important role in reducing mental and physical stresses. Trial participants who were given magnesium, zinc, and calcium experienced dramatic decreases in psychological distress.

Summer Peaches and Parsley

This combination has refreshing summery flavors and provides a substantial source of mood-altering essential amino acids from the protein powder and the hulled hemp seeds.

Serves 2

SMOOTHIE

1 cup sliced peach

1 cup carrot juice

2 large lettuce leaves

1/4 cup protein powder

Combine all the ingredients in a blender and blend until smooth.

TOPPINGS

1/2 cup chopped peach

2 tablespoons hulled hemp seeds

Sprigs of fresh flat-leaf parsley leaves

Pour the smoothie into two small bowls and sprinkle each with half of the toppings and serve.

NUTRITION FACTS (GRAMS PER SERVING)
Calories 183, Fat 3, Protein 16, Carbs 20, Fiber 3, NetCarbs 17

Deregulation of neurotransmitters affects mood, anxiety, and the ability to manage stress. Amino acids are the building blocks the body uses to make neurotransmitters and daily intake can increase serotonin and dopamine while decreasing stress hormones, such as cortisol.

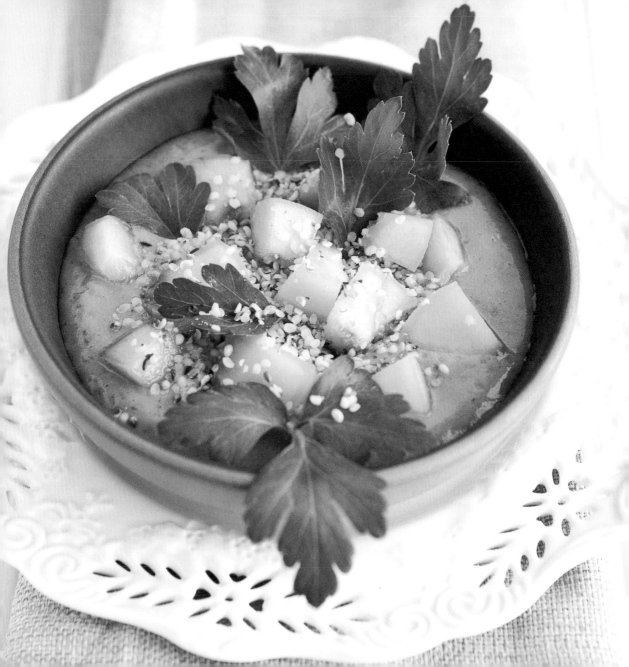

Parsley Apple Crunch

This fresh bowl is loaded with fiber, flavonoids, and essential fatty acids that promote weight loss and help prevent weight gain.

Serves 2

SMOOTHIE	TOPPINGS
1 cup sliced Fuji apple	$1/2$ cup raspberries
1 cup fresh flat-leaf parsley leaves	$1/2$ cup chopped apple
1 cup raspberries	2 tablespoons toasted hulled hemp seeds
$1/2$ cup carrot juice	

Combine all the ingredients in a blender and blend until smooth.

Pour the smoothie into two small bowls and sprinkle each with half of the toppings and serve.

NUTRITION FACTS (GRAMS PER SERVING)
Calories 170, Fat 5, Protein 6, Carbs 31, Fiber 4, NetCarbs 27

Intake of high-flavonoid foods, such as apples, parsley, bananas, peaches, blueberries, and romaine lettuce, help prevent weight gain.

Garden Berry

This bowl is tart and sweet, and rich in flavonoids from leafy chard and loads of berries.

Serves 2

SMOOTHIE

1 cup fresh chard leaves
1 cup blackberries
1 cup strawberry halves
$1/4$ cup chia seeds
$1/4$ cup black currant juice

Combine all the ingredients in a blender and blend until smooth.

TOPPINGS

$1/2$ cup blackberries
2 tablespoons pomegranate arils
2 tablespoons hulled hemp seeds

Pour the smoothie into two small bowls and sprinkle each with half of the toppings and serve.

NUTRITION FACTS (GRAMS PER SERVING)
Calories 249, Fat 13, Protein 11, Carbs 31, Fiber 19, NetCarbs 12

Daily intake of fruits and vegetables promote weight loss and lower the risk of developing cardiovascular diseases and cancers. Plant fiber acts as a prebiotic, feeding the probiotics in the GI tract. Probiotics are living organisms that produce protective compounds that provide significant protection against our most common degenerative diseases.

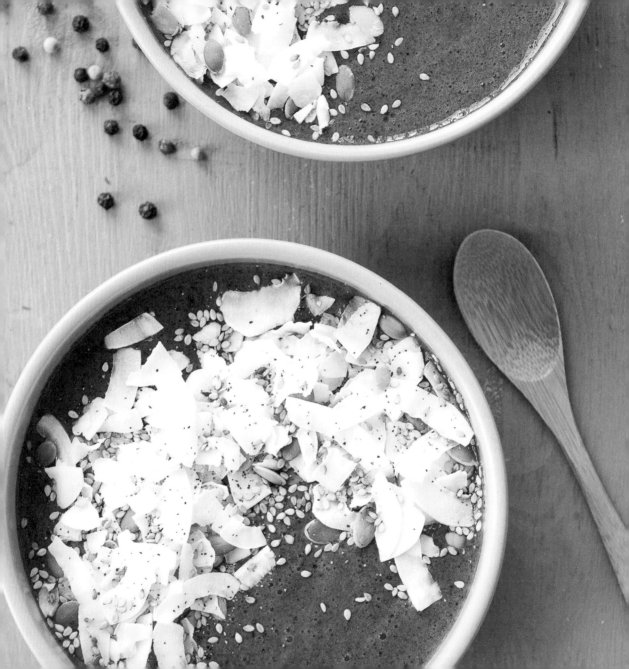

Blueberry Cherry Whip

This bowl is a creamy, deep purple blend that's rich in minerals and beneficial probiotics. The toppings of pumpkin and sesame seeds provide antiaging zinc.

Serves 2

SMOOTHIE

1 (1-inch) piece turmeric root, peeled and minced

1 cup blueberries

1 cup pitted dark sweet cherries

1 cup coconut milk yogurt

1/2 cup fresh spinach leaves

Combine all the ingredients in a blender and blend until smooth.

TOPPINGS

2 tablespoons pumpkin seeds

2 tablespoons unsweetened flaked coconut

2 teaspoons sesame seeds

Pinch of freshly ground black pepper

Pour the smoothie into two small bowls and sprinkle each with half of the toppings and serve.

NUTRITION FACTS (GRAMS PER SERVING)
Calories 190, Fat 9 Protein 6, Carbs 22, Fiber 4, NetCarbs 18

Zinc is an essential mineral necessary for immune function, as well as the regulation of blood sugar and inflammation.

Ginger Grapefruit Warmer

Pleasantly warming, this bowl has sweet and tangy
ingredients that help to regulate blood sugar and increase weight loss.

Serves 2

SMOOTHIE

2 cups grapefruit segments

1 (1-inch) piece ginger root,
peeled and minced

1 cup sliced apple

1 cup fresh spinach leaves

$1/4$ cup carrot juice

$1/4$ cup chia seeds

Pinch of cayenne pepper

Combine all the ingredients in
a blender and blend until smooth.

TOPPINGS

$1/2$ cup chopped apple

$1/2$ cup shredded carrot

2 tablespoons chopped pistachios

Pour the smoothie into two small
bowls and sprinkle each with half
of the toppings and serve.

NUTRITION FACTS (GRAMS PER SERVING)
Calories 220, Fat 12, Protein 8, Carbs 28, Fiber 14, NetCarbs 14

Chia seeds, grapefruit, and apple each provide nutrients that boost weight loss by
decreasing body fat, stabilizing blood sugar, and reducing inflammation.

Sweet Greens

This creamy bowl has bright peach flavor and
provides potent amounts of protein and essential fatty acids.

Serves 2

SMOOTHIE

$^1/_2$ avocado, pitted and peeled

2 cups fresh spinach leaves

1 cup sliced peach

1 cup almond milk

$^1/_4$ cup hulled hemp seeds

$^1/_4$ cup protein powder

Combine all the ingredients in
a blender and blend until smooth.

TOPPINGS

$^1/_2$ cup blueberries

$^1/_2$ cup chopped peach

2 tablespoons sliced almonds

Pour the smoothie into two
small bowls and divide the
toppings over each and serve.

NUTRITION FACTS (GRAMS PER SERVING)
Calories 341, Fat 13, Protein 21, Carbs 31, Fiber 10, NetCarbs 21

Hulled hemp seeds provide omega-3 fatty acids and 3 grams of protein per tablespoon.
The protein powder adds an additional 7 to 24 grams of protein per tablespoon, depending on the product. Avocados add healthful fats that help reduce cholesterol levels and they provide 35 percent more potassium than a banana as well as vitamins B_5, B_6, C, E, and K.

Vanilla Basil Whip

This bowl is light and creamy and has a savory herbal fragrance.

Serves 2

SMOOTHIE	TOPPINGS
1/2 avocado, pitted and peeled	2 tablespoons sliced almonds
1 cup fresh basil leaves	Sprigs of fresh basil leaves
1 cup almond milk	Sprigs of fresh thyme leaves
1/4 cup hulled hemp seeds	6 rice crackers
2 teaspoons pure vanilla extract, or 2 vanilla beans (optional)	

Combine all the ingredients in a blender and blend until smooth.

Pour the smoothie into two small bowls and sprinkle each with half of the almonds, basil, and thyme and serve with the rice crackers on the side.

NUTRITION FACTS (GRAMS PER SERVING)
Calories 220, Fat 10, Protein 7, Carbs 10, Fiber 5, NetCarbs 5

The nutrients in avocados, including essential fatty acids, fiber, potassium, magnesium, folate, vitamin B_6, niacin, pantothenic acid, riboflavin, choline, lutein, zeaxanthin, and phytosterols, support cardiovascular health, weight management, and healthy aging.

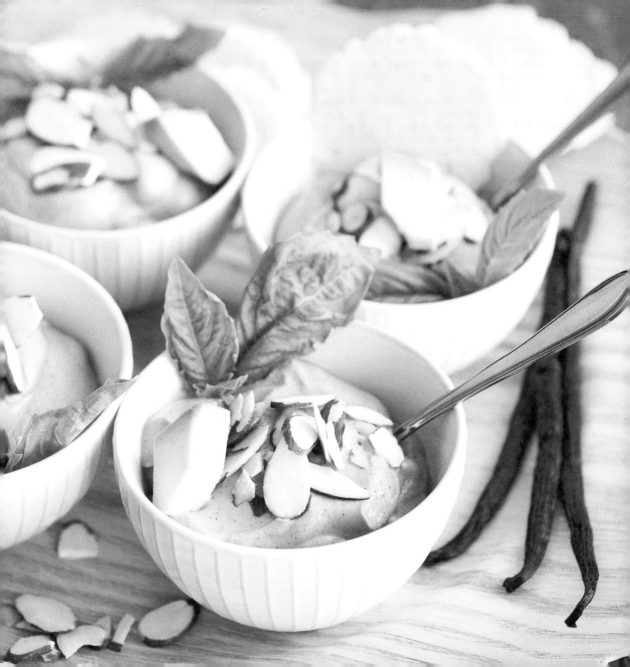

Banana Protein Crunch

This green bowl is rich in protein and fiber,
and topped with fresh sweet berries and a light almond crunch.

Serves 2

SMOOTHIE

1 banana, peeled

2 cups fresh spinach leaves

1 cup almond milk

$1/4$ cup hulled hemp seeds

$1/4$ cup protein powder

1 teaspoon ground turmeric

Combine all the ingredients in a blender and blend until smooth.

TOPPINGS

$1/2$ cup sliced strawberries

$1/2$ cup peeled, sliced banana

2 tablespoons sliced almonds

Pour the smoothie into two small bowls and add half of the toppings to each and serve.

NUTRITION FACTS (GRAMS PER SERVING)
Calories 303, Fat 12, Protein 22, Carbs 28, Fiber 6, NetCarbs 22

Strawberries are low on the glycemic index because they contain beta-glucans, a natural soluble fiber that slows the absorption of carbohydrates.

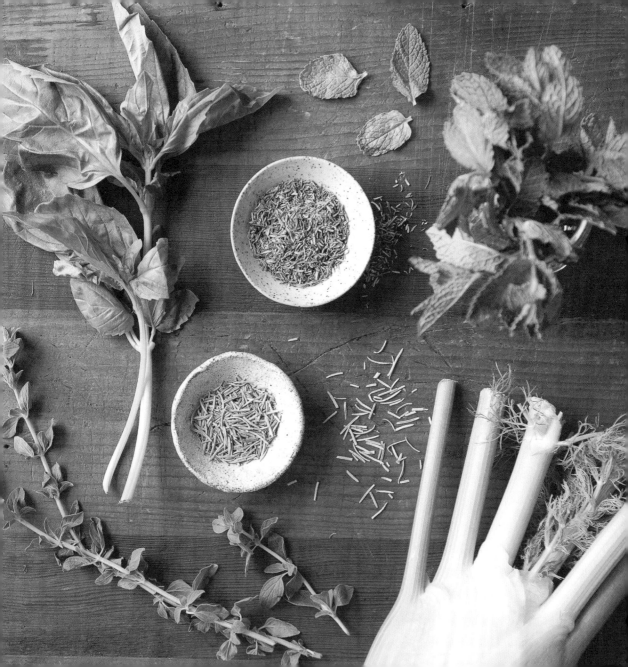

CHAPTER
5
HERB
BOWL
RECIPES

Cantaloupe Basil Cooler

This refreshing blend has cool cucumber and melon flavor, with immune-boosting and pain-moderating effects.

Serves 2

SMOOTHIE

1 cup orange segments
$^1/_2$ cantaloupe, without rind
1 cup fresh basil leaves
1 cup peeled, sliced cucumber
$^1/_4$ cup hulled hemp seeds
3 tablespoons black cherry juice concentrate

Combine all the ingredients in a blender and blend until smooth.

TOPPINGS

2 tablespoons pomegranate arils
2 tablespoons hulled hemp seeds
Sprigs of fresh basil leaves

Pour the smoothie into two small bowls and sprinkle each with half of the toppings and serve.

NUTRITION FACTS (GRAMS PER SERVING)
Calories 196, Fat 9, Protein 9, Carbs 19, Fiber 5, NetCarbs 14

Basil contains a natural compound called linalool that has antioxidant, pain-reducing, neuroprotective, antiviral, and antibacterial activity.

Creamy Cilantro and Citrus

This green blend has subtle herb, citrus, and tropical flavors.
Cilantro seeds, which are known as coriander, provide powerful
medicinal effects against a range of common degenerative health conditions.

Serves 2

SMOOTHIE

1/2 avocado, pitted and peeled

1/4 lime with peel, chopped
(seeds removed)

1 cup fresh cilantro leaves

1 cup peeled, sliced cucumber

1/4 cup coconut milk beverage

Combine all the ingredients in
a blender and blend until smooth.

TOPPINGS

1/2 cup peeled, sliced cucumber

2 teaspoons sesame seeds

2 teaspoons coriander seeds

Sprigs of fresh cilantro leaves

Pour the smoothie into two small
bowls and sprinkle each with half of
the toppings and serve.

NUTRITION FACTS (GRAMS PER SERVING)
Calories 100, Fat 7, Protein 3, Carbs 7, Fiber 4, NetCarbs 3

Cilantro provides antimicrobial, antioxidant, hypoglycemic, hypolipidemic, analgesic, anti-inflammatory, anticonvulsant, and anticancer benefits as well as protection against Alzheimer's disease. Additionally, the coriander seeds provide proven benefits for those with asthma and bronchiolitis.

Oregano Citrus Power

This bright orange bowl has carrot and citrus flavors
with fragrant oregano that provide phytochemicals to protect
against inflammation and fight bacterial infections.

Serves 2

SMOOTHIE

2 cups tangerine segments

1 cup cantaloupe, without rind

$1/4$ cup carrot juice

$1/4$ cup hulled hemp seeds

2 tablespoons tangerine zest

1 tablespoon fresh oregano leaves

Combine all the ingredients in
a blender and blend until smooth.

TOPPINGS

$1/2$ cup chopped cantaloupe,
without rind

2 teaspoons sliced almonds

2 teaspoons hulled hemp seeds

Sprigs of fresh oregano leaves

Pour the smoothie into two small
bowls and sprinkle each with half
of the toppings and serve.

NUTRITION FACTS (GRAMS PER SERVING)
Calories 219, Fat 10, Protein 9, Carbs 24, Fiber 6, NetCarbs 18

Oregano contains powerful compounds, such as carvacrol, cymene, linalool, and terpinene, which reduce inflammation, kill bacteria and fungus, and have antiproliferative activity against human cancer cells.

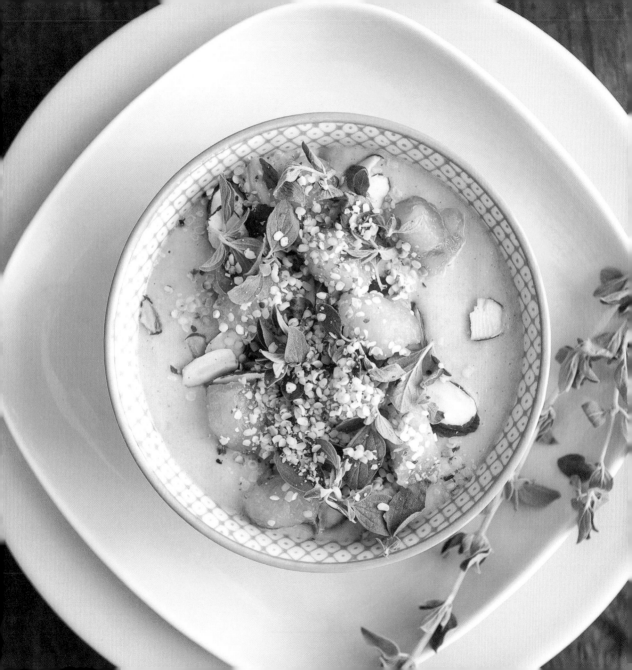

Cherry Insomnia Elixir

This blend of melatonin-rich whole foods contains powerful compounds that support sleep. Toppings of tart kiwi, walnuts, and banana boost the insomnia-ending effects even further.

Serves 2

SMOOTHIE

1 kiwi, peeled

$^1/_2$ banana, peeled

1 cup pitted dark sweet cherries

1 cup lettuce

$^1/_4$ cup chia seeds

3 tablespoons black cherry juice concentrate

2 tablespoons chopped banana peel

Combine all the ingredients in a blender and blend until smooth.

TOPPINGS

$^1/_2$ cup peeled, sliced banana

$^1/_2$ cup peeled, sliced kiwi

2 tablespoons chopped walnuts

Sprigs of fresh thyme leaves

Pour the smoothie into two small bowls and sprinkle each with half of the toppings and serve.

NUTRITION FACTS (GRAMS PER SERVING)
Calories 310, Fat 16, Protein 9, Carbs 42, Fiber 17, Net Carbs 25

Lettuce, cherry, kiwi, and walnut are all functional foods that contain nutrients and compounds, including tryptophan, GABA, calcium, potassium, melatonin, pyridoxine, ornithine, and hexadecanoic acid, which modulate the neurochemical factors that affect sleep.

Rosemary Peach Forget-Me-Not

This bowl has a fresh, herbal fragrance and tree-fruit sweetness.
All of the ingredients in this powerful medicinal blend support memory
by reducing oxidation and inflammation in the brain and digestive tract.

Serves 2

SMOOTHIE
1 cup lettuce

1 cup sliced apple

$1/2$ cup sliced peach

$1/2$ cup fresh mint leaves

3 tablespoons black cherry juice concentrate

1 (1-inch) piece turmeric root, peeled and minced

1 teaspoon ground rosemary

Combine all the ingredients in a blender and blend until smooth.

TOPPINGS
$1/2$ cup chopped apple

$1/2$ cup cherry halves

Sprigs of fresh mint leaves

Pour the smoothie into two small
bowls and sprinkle each with half
of the toppings and serve.

NUTRITION FACTS (GRAMS PER SERVING)
Calories 100, Fat 0, Protein 2, Carbs 25, Fiber 4, NetCarbs 21

Rosemary contains phenolic antioxidants with therapeutic benefits in Alzheimer's
treatment, as they reduce brain inflammation and amyloid formation, as well as provide
general antioxidant-mediated neuronal protection.

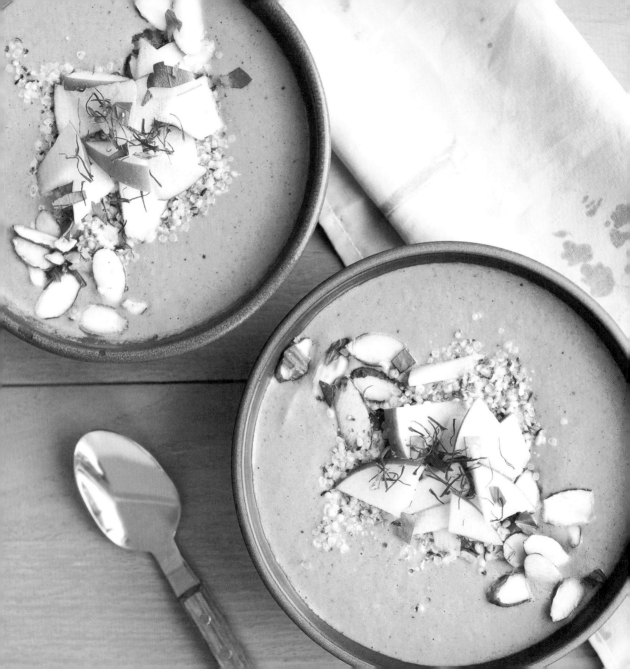

Creamy Vanilla Parsley

This bowl has sweet apples, rich vanilla, and bright parsley.

Serves 2

SMOOTHIE

1 cup fresh flat-leaf parsley leaves

2 cups sliced apple

$^1/_2$ cup vanilla almond milk

$^1/_4$ cup hulled hemp seeds

2 teaspoons pure vanilla extract

Combine all the ingredients in a blender and blend until smooth.

TOPPINGS

$^1/_2$ cup chopped apple

2 teaspoons sliced almonds

2 teaspoons hulled hemp seeds

Sprigs of fresh flat-leaf parsley leaves

Pinch of saffron threads

Pour the smoothie into two small bowls and sprinkle each with half of the toppings and serve.

NUTRITION FACTS (GRAMS PER SERVING)
Calories 260, Fat 14, Protein 12, Carbs 24, Fiber 7, NetCarbs 17

Flat-leaf, or Italian, parsley contains apegenin flavonoids that inhibit blood clots and platelet aggregation, helping reduce the risk for stroke.

Avocado Basil Whip

This creamy, savory bowl is perfect as an appetizer or savory dessert for a healthy dinner party. Packed with herbs, this blend provides anti-inflammatory and antioxidant benefits.

Serves 4

SMOOTHIE

1/2 avocado, pitted and peeled

1 (1-inch) piece turmeric root, peeled and minced

1 cup fresh basil leaves

1 cup coconut milk yogurt

1 tablespoon fresh oregano leaves

1 teaspoon ground rosemary

Pinch of freshly ground black pepper

Combine all the ingredients in a blender and blend until smooth.

TOPPINGS

2 tablespoons sliced almonds

Sprigs of fresh oregano leaves

Pinch of freshly ground black pepper

8 black pepper rice crackers

Pour the smoothie into four small bowls and sprinkle each with one quarter of the almonds, oregano, and black pepper. Serve the rice crackers on the side.

NUTRITION FACTS (GRAMS PER SERVING)
Calories 107, Fat 7, Protein 3, Carbs 9, Fiber 4, Net Carbs 5

Oregano, rosemary, and turmeric have polyphenolic antioxidants with antimicrobial action against bacterial and fungal infections, such as acne, toenail fungus, and strep.

Blueberry Spearmint

This fragrant bowl has sweet and savory notes with healthful mint, which has been found to help improve pain and stiffness in the body.

Serves 2

SMOOTHIE

1 banana, peeled
1 cup fresh spearmint leaves
1 cup blueberries
$1/2$ cup almond milk
$1/4$ cup chia seeds
$1/4$ cup protein powder

Combine all the ingredients in a blender and blend until smooth.

TOPPINGS

$1/2$ cup blueberries
$1/2$ cup peeled sliced banana
2 tablespoons sliced almonds
Sprigs of fresh mint leaves

Pour the smoothie into two small bowls and sprinkle each with half of the toppings and serve.

NUTRITION FACTS (GRAMS PER SERVING)
Calories 350, Fat 14, Protein 19, Carbs 45, Fiber 18, Net Carbs 27

Spearmint is rich in rosmarinic acid, which can significantly improve the stiffness and pain of osteoarthritis, when ingested daily. Blueberries reduce the inflammation that promotes insulin resistance, thus providing some protection against metabolic syndrome, diabetes, and hypoglycemia.

Fennel Berry Sorbet

This beautiful magenta blend has fresh, nutrient-rich foods
that provide protection from the damaging effects of high blood sugar levels.
This delicious blend is topped with crunchy pistachios for their healthy fats.

Serves 2

SMOOTHIE

2 cups blood orange segments

1 cup raspberries

1/2 cup chopped fennel bulb

1/4 cup chia seeds

3 tablespoons black cherry
juice concentrate

2 teaspoons coriander seeds

Combine all the ingredients in
a blender and blend until smooth.

TOPPINGS

2 tablespoons chopped pistachios

Sprigs of chopped fennel greens

Pour the smoothie into two small
bowls and sprinkle each with half
of the toppings and serve.

NUTRITION FACTS (GRAMS PER SERVING)
Calories 302, Fat 12, Protein 11, Carbs 46, Fiber 20, NetCarbs 26

Children and adolescents with type 1 diabetes who consume more fruits and vegetables,
such as blood oranges, greens, berries, and herbs, have a lower incidence of microvascular disease, such as retinopathy, later in life.

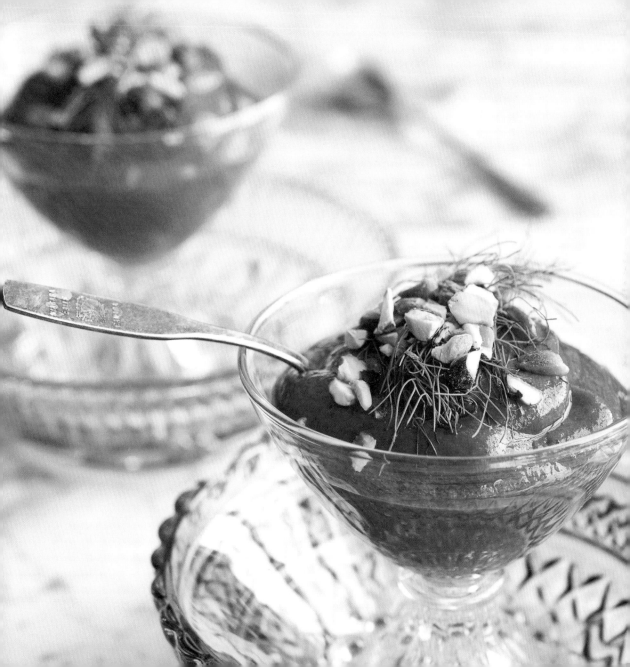

Strawberry Thyme Soother

This herbal bowl is balanced with thyme and fragrant strawberries. Compounds in thyme have been shown to support recovery from common ailments, such as cold and flu.

Serves 2

SMOOTHIE

1 banana, peeled

1 cup strawberry halves

$1/2$ cup almond milk

$1/4$ cup hulled hemp seeds

2 tablespoons fresh thyme leaves

Combine all the ingredients in a blender and blend until smooth.

TOPPINGS

$1/2$ cup sliced strawberry halves

2 tablespoons toasted hulled hemp seeds

2 teaspoons fresh thyme leaves

Pour the smoothie into two small bowls and sprinkle each with half of the toppings and serve.

NUTRITION FACTS (GRAMS PER SERVING)
Calories 196, Fat 10, Protein 8, Carbs 18, Fiber 5, NetCarbs 13

Both fresh and dried thyme contain rosmarinic acid, ursolic acid, oleanolic acid, and thymoquinol, which support recovery from viruses, stomachache, cough, and infections.

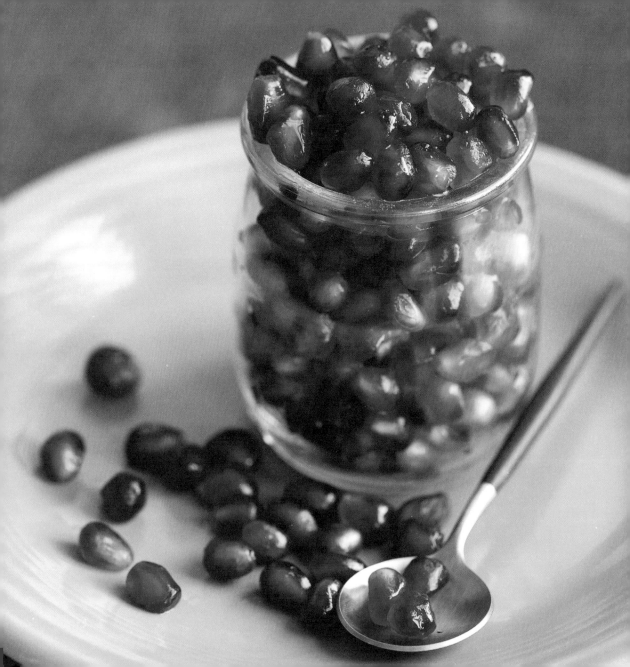

CHAPTER 6

POMEGRANATE BOWL RECIPES

Mango Pom Refresher

This tropical bowl has fresh turmeric scent and sweet pomegranate flavor.

Serves 2

SMOOTHIE

1 (1-inch) piece turmeric root, peeled and minced

1 cup pitted and peeled mango

1/2 cup pomegranate juice concentrate

1/4 cup chia seeds

Pinch of freshly ground black pepper

Combine all the ingredients in a blender and blend until smooth.

TOPPINGS

2 tablespoons pomegranate arils

2 tablespoons toasted hulled hemp seeds

Sprigs of fresh mint leaves

Pour the smoothie into two small bowls and sprinkle each with half of the toppings and serve.

NUTRITION FACTS (GRAMS PER SERVING)
Calories 250, Fat 12, Protein 10, Carbs 31, Fiber 14, NetCarbs 17

Pomegranates have a long-standing superfood reputation, as their seeds, called arils, contain concentrated amounts of highly active antioxidant nutrients.

Tangerine Pomegranate Sorbet

This fruity and potent blend is packed with ascorbic acid that supports production of collagen to help firm and protect the skin from environmental damage.

Serves 4

SMOOTHIE

1 cup tangerine segments
1 (1-inch) piece turmeric root, peeled and minced
1 cup strawberry halves
1 cup pitted dark sweet cherries
1/4 cup pomegranate juice concentrate
1/4 cup chia seeds
Pinch of freshly ground black pepper

Combine all the ingredients in a blender and blend until smooth.

TOPPINGS

1/2 cup peeled, sliced banana
1/4 cup cherry halves
2 tablespoons pomegranate arils

Pour the smoothie into four small bowls and sprinkle each with one quarter of the toppings and serve.

NUTRITION FACTS (GRAMS PER SERVING)
Calories 120, Fat 5, Protein 4 , Carbs 18 Fiber 8, NetCarbs 10

Pomegranate juice is rich in vitamin C and coumaric acid. These naturally occurring antioxidants enhance collagen growth and inhibit the development of age spots.

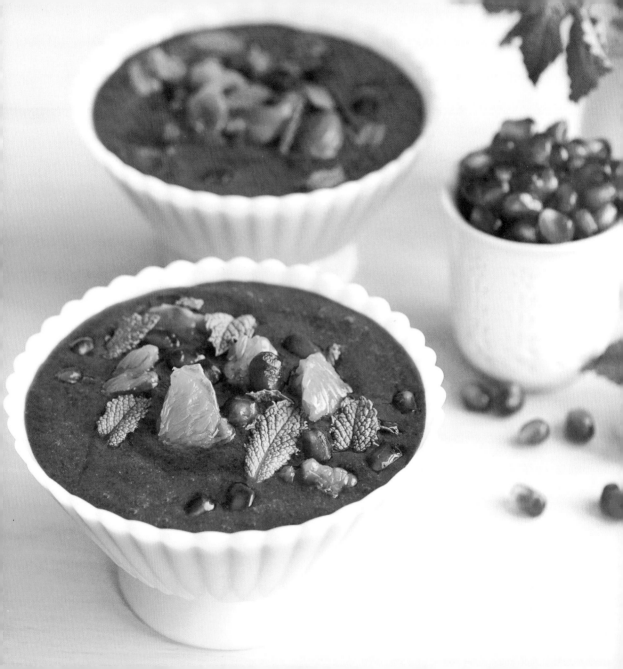

Pomegranate Tangerine Crush

The blueberries, citrus, and pomegranate in this sorbet-like bowl all contain high levels of antioxidants that help protect the skin from the sun's harmful rays.

Serves 2

SMOOTHIE

1 cup tangerine segments

$1/2$ banana, peeled

1 cup wild blueberries

$1/4$ cup hulled hemp seeds

3 tablespoons pomegranate juice concentrate

2 tablespoons tangerine zest

Combine all the ingredients in a blender and blend until smooth.

TOPPINGS

2 tablespoons minced tangerine segments

2 tablespoons pomegranate arils

Sprigs of fresh mint leaves

Pour the smoothie into two small bowls and sprinkle each with half of the toppings and serve.

NUTRITION FACTS (GRAMS PER SERVING)
Calories 175, Fat 6, Protein 7, Carbs 20, Fiber 8, Net Carbs 12

Blueberries are rich in antioxidants, and wild blueberries contain up to ten times the concentration of antioxidants found in cultivated berries.

Wild Berry Pom

This bright bowl delivers fresh turmeric and fruit flavor.
Turmeric provides the powerful antioxidant curcumin.

Serves 2

SMOOTHIE

1 (1-inch) piece turmeric root, peeled and minced

1 cup wild blueberries

1 cup fresh spinach leaves

1/4 cup hulled hemp seeds

3 tablespoons pomegranate juice concentrate

Pinch of freshly ground black pepper

Combine all the ingredients in a blender and blend until smooth.

TOPPINGS

2 tablespoons hulled hemp seeds

2 tablespoons pomegranate arils

Pinch of freshly ground black pepper

Pour the smoothie into two small bowls and sprinkle each with half of the toppings and serve.

NUTRITION FACTS (GRAMS PER SERVING)
Calories 222, Fat 9, Protein 10, Carbs 22, Fiber 7, NetCarbs 15

Curcumin, found in turmeric, has proven anti-inflammatory, immunomodulatory, and anticancer effects. It is a powerful nutrient that protects women against UTIs (urinary tract infections) and other infections of the female genital tract, including vaginal infections and gynecologic cancers.

Cranberry Ginger Warmer

This healing bowl pairs sweet strawberries
and tart cranberries with turmeric and ginger.

Serves 2

SMOOTHIE

1 (1-inch) piece turmeric root,
peeled and minced

1 (1-inch) piece ginger root,
peeled and minced

1 cup strawberry halves

1/2 cup pitted dark sweet cherries

1/4 cup fresh cranberries

1/4 cup protein powder

3 tablespoons pomegranate
juice concentrate

Combine all the ingredients in
a blender and blend until smooth.

TOPPINGS

2 tablespoons pomegranate arils

2 tablespoons chopped cashews

2 tablespoons chopped hazelnuts

Pour the smoothie into two small
bowls and sprinkle each with half
of the toppings and serve.

NUTRITION FACTS (GRAMS PER SERVING)
Calories 229, Fat 8, Protein 16, Carbs 23, Fiber 5, NetCarbs 18

Vegetable-based protein powders, such as pea, soy, hemp, and rice, as well as powders
from nuts and seeds, contain fiber that improve weight control in overweight and obese
adults via gut-mediated changes in metabolic health.

Golden Granola Powerhouse

This protein-packed bowl has sweet fruit flavor
and powerful antioxidants from turmeric root.

Serves 2

SMOOTHIE

1 banana, peeled

1 (1-inch) piece turmeric root,
peeled and minced

1 cup sliced peach

$1/4$ cup protein powder

3 tablespoons pomegranate
juice concentrate

Pinch of freshly ground black pepper

Combine all the ingredients in
a blender and blend until smooth.

TOPPINGS

$1/2$ cup peeled, sliced banana

$1/2$ cup chopped peach

$1/4$ cup pumpkin seeds

2 tablespoons granola

Pour the smoothie into two small
bowls and sprinkle each with half
of the toppings and serve.

NUTRITION FACTS (GRAMS PER SERVING)
Calories 286, Fat 8, Protein 18, Carbs 35, Fiber 6, NetCarbs 29

Turmeric is a well-known anti-inflammatory, antioxidant, and antilipidemic that provides protection from many conditions, such as neurocognitive disorders, obesity, diabetes, and cancers.

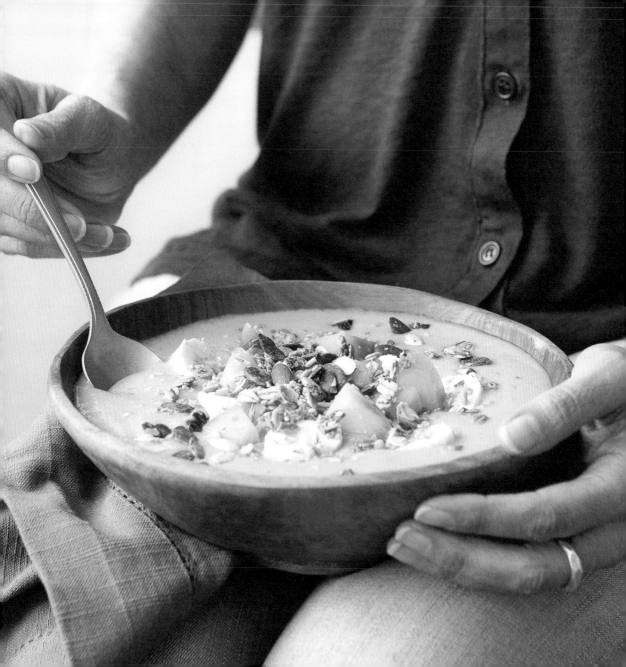

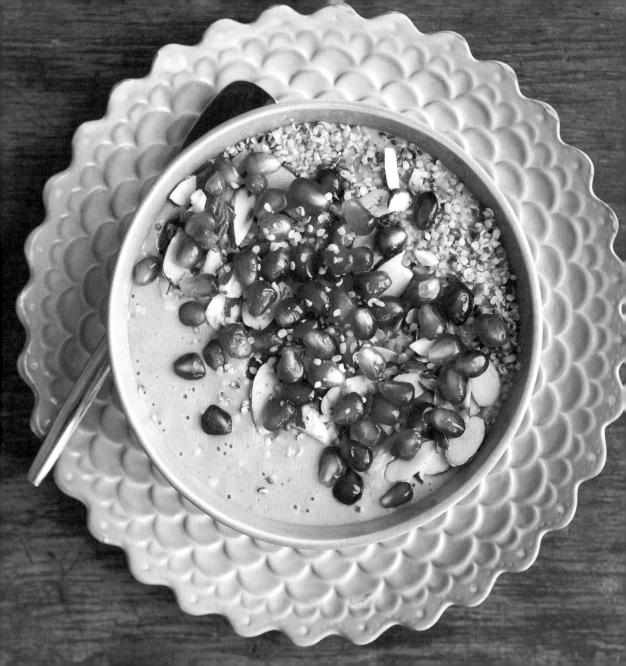

Almond Banana Crunch

This simple blend has a powerful weight-loss combination.
High levels of protein and fiber provide long-lasting satiation.
It is topped with almonds and pomegranate seeds for a satisfying crunch.

Serves 2

SMOOTHIE

2 bananas, peeled

1 (1-inch) piece turmeric root, peeled and minced

1/2 cup almond milk

1/4 cup hulled hemp seeds

1/4 cup protein powder

Combine all the ingredients in a blender and blend until smooth.

TOPPINGS

2 tablespoons pomegranate arils

2 tablespoons sliced almonds

2 tablespoons hulled hemp seeds

Pour the smoothie into two small bowls and sprinkle each with half of the toppings and serve.

NUTRITION FACTS (GRAMS PER SERVING)
Calories 304, Fat 10, Protein 21, Carbs 30, Fiber 6, NetCarbs 23

Nuts and seeds contain antioxidants, fiber, and catechins, which are metabolized by the microbes in the colon, creating compounds that support weight loss and provide cancer protection.

Strawberry Apricot Pom

This bright blend has flavors reminiscent of a summer garden.

Serves 2

SMOOTHIE

1 apricot, halved and pitted

2 cups strawberry halves

$^1/_2$ cup fresh Swiss chard leaves

$^1/_4$ cup pomegranate juice

$^1/_4$ cup hulled hemp seeds

Combine all the ingredients in a blender and blend until smooth.

TOPPINGS

$^1/_2$ cup sliced strawberries

2 tablespoons pomegranate arils

2 tablespoons hulled hemp seeds

Pour the smoothie into two small bowls and sprinkle each with half of the toppings and serve.

NUTRITION FACTS (GRAMS PER SERVING)
Calories 254, Fat 11, Protein 9, Carbs 28, Fiber 17, Net Carbs 11

Pomegranate seeds and juice provide concentrated antioxidants and bioactive polyphenols that not only provide anti-inflammatory, antiaging, and chemopreventive effects, but also neutralize free radicals and the damaging effects of some environmental toxins.

Creamy Berry Pomegranate

Tart pomegranate and nutty pumpkin seeds blend together to
provide vitamin C and zinc for improved immunity in this berry bowl.

Serves 2

SMOOTHIE

1 banana, peeled

1 cup blackberries

$1/4$ cup hulled hemp seeds

$1/4$ cup pumpkin seeds

3 tablespoons pomegranate
juice concentrate

Combine all the ingredients in
a blender and blend until smooth.

TOPPINGS

$1/4$ cup pomegranate arils

2 tablespoons pumpkin seeds

2 tablespoons sliced almonds

Pour the smoothie into two
small bowls and sprinkle each
with half of the toppings and serve.

NUTRITION FACTS (GRAMS PER SERVING)
Calories 384 Fat 24, Protein 14, Carbs 32, Fiber 12 , NetCarbs 20

Pumpkin seeds are one of our richest vegan food sources of the mineral zinc, which modulates immunity, decreases incidence of infections and oxidative stress, and acts as an anti-inflammatory agent. Zinc also supports insulin function, which can lead to fewer sugar cravings.

Peaches and Cream

This creamy and tart bowl is topped with crunchy walnuts and pomegranate arils. The coconut milk yogurt and probiotic powder supply beneficial probiotics for gut health and weight management while the banana provides the prebiotics needed for the microbes to thrive.

Serves 2

SMOOTHIE

1 cup sliced peach

$1/2$ cup blueberries

$1/2$ cup coconut milk yogurt

$1/4$ cup hulled hemp seeds

3 tablespoons pomegranate juice concentrate

1 teaspoon probiotic powder

Combine all the ingredients in a blender and blend until smooth.

TOPPINGS

$1/2$ cup peeled, sliced banana

$1/4$ cup pomegranate arils

2 tablespoons chopped walnuts

Pour the smoothie into two small bowls and sprinkle each with half of the toppings and serve.

NUTRITION FACTS (GRAMS PER SERVING)
Calories 223, Fat 8, Protein 8, Carbs 30, Fiber 8, NetCarbs 22

Lactobacilli, a specific and common microbial strain, increases butyric acid in the GI tract, where it promotes weight loss and protects the GI tract from diverticulitis and cancer development.

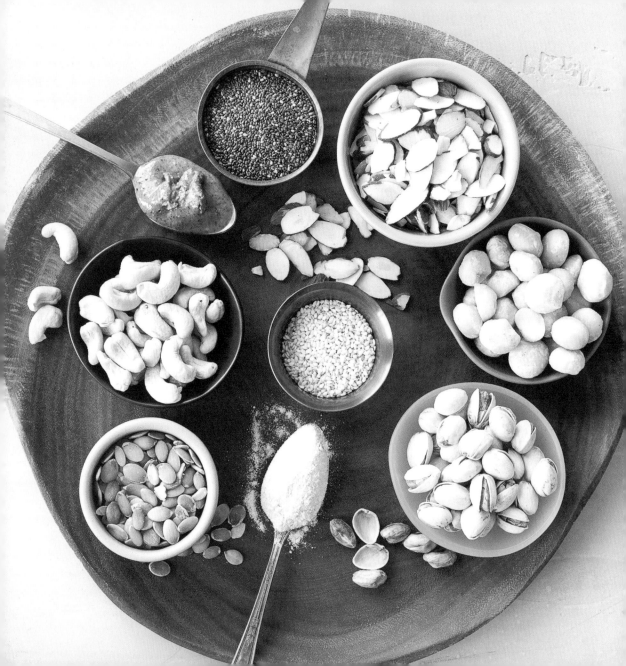

POWER BOWL RECIPES

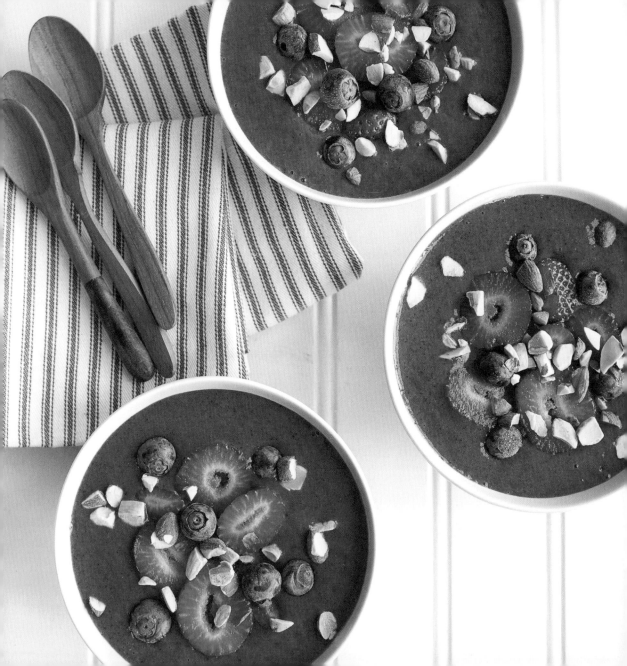

Kid-Friendly Blend

This creamy, high-protein bowl is topped with crunchy and sweet treats, making it satisfying for picky eaters.

Serves 4

SMOOTHIE

$1/2$ banana, peeled

$1/2$ cup blueberries

$1/2$ cup pitted dark sweet cherries

2 large lettuce leaves

$1/4$ cup almond milk

2 tablespoons hulled hemp seeds

2 tablespoons protein powder

Combine all the ingredients in a blender and blend until smooth.

TOPPINGS

$1/4$ cup sliced strawberries

$1/4$ cup blueberries

1 tablespoon sliced almonds

Pour the smoothie into four small bowls and sprinkle each with one quarter of the toppings and serve.

NUTRITION FACTS (GRAMS PER SERVING)
Calories 212, Fat 6, Protein 12, Carbs 26, Fiber 6, Net Carbs 20

Almonds are a rich source of vitamin E, protein, fiber, B vitamins, minerals, and healthful fats. They also provide phytosterols, which help lower cholesterol levels.

Maternity Power Bowl

This soothing blend is creamy, nutty, and full of protein.
Spinach is an excellent source of vital folate. Essential amino acids
support the growth of new life, and turmeric soothes inflammation.

Serves 2

SMOOTHIE

2 bananas, peeled

1 (1-inch) piece turmeric root,
peeled and minced

1 cup fresh spinach leaves

1 cup hemp milk

$1/4$ cup protein powder

$1/4$ cup toasted hulled hemp seeds

2 tablespoons nut butter

Pinch of freshly ground black pepper

Combine all the ingredients in
a blender and blend until smooth.

TOPPINGS

$1/2$ cup sliced strawberries

$1/2$ cup blueberries

2 tablespoons sunflower seeds

2 tablespoons toasted hulled
hemp seeds

Pour the smoothie into two small
bowls and sprinkle each with half
of the toppings and serve.

NUTRITION FACTS (GRAMS PER SERVING)
Calories 494, Fat 20, Protein 27, Carbs 49, Fiber 10, NetCarbs 39

Consistent intake of amino acids, essential fatty acids, and B vitamins are needed throughout pregnancy to reduce risk for the development of hyperglycemia, hyper-insulinemia,
hyperlipidemia, hypertension, and insulin resistance.

Athlete's Power Bowl

This rich bowl has the anti-inflammatory benefits of turmeric root, the mood improving benefits of oils from avocado, and energizing amino acids from the protein powder and hulled hemp seeds.

Serves 2

SMOOTHIE

1 banana, peeled

1/2 avocado, pitted and peeled

1 (1-inch) piece turmeric root, peeled and minced

1/2 cup raspberries

1/2 cup hemp milk

1/4 cup hulled hemp seeds

1/4 cup protein powder

1/4 cup chia seeds

Pinch of freshly ground black pepper

Combine all the ingredients in a blender and blend until smooth.

TOPPINGS

2 tablespoons chopped pecans

2 tablespoons pumpkin seeds

2 teaspoons sesame seeds

Pour the smoothie into two small bowls and sprinkle each with half of the toppings and serve.

NUTRITION FACTS (GRAMS PER SERVING)
Calories 551, Fat 33, Protein 28, Carbs 41, Fiber 21, NetCarbs 20

Increasing manganese intake through such foods as pumpkin seeds, pecans, and sesame seeds has a positive effect on blood pressure.

Coconut Berry Cream

This vibrant bowl blends antioxidant-rich blueberries with
essential amino acids provided by the protein powder.

Serves 2

SMOOTHIE

2 cups blueberries

1/2 cup coconut milk beverage

1/4 cup pumpkin seeds

1/4 cup protein powder

Combine all the ingredients in
a blender and blend until smooth.

TOPPINGS

2 tablespoons blueberries

2 tablespoons unsweetened
flaked coconut

2 tablespoons pumpkin seeds

Pour the smoothie into two small
bowls and sprinkle each with half
of the toppings and serve.

NUTRITION FACTS (GRAMS PER SERVING)
Calories 361, Fat 15, Protein 20, Carbs 27, Fiber 11, Net Carbs 16

Protein-rich foods, such as nuts, seeds, and protein powders, contain the amino acids
that are the building blocks for the production of neurotransmitters that manage mood
and pain. A diet rich in amino acids ensures a constant supply of the materials needed to
make adequate amounts of the chemicals that give us feelings of contentment, relaxation, and satiety.

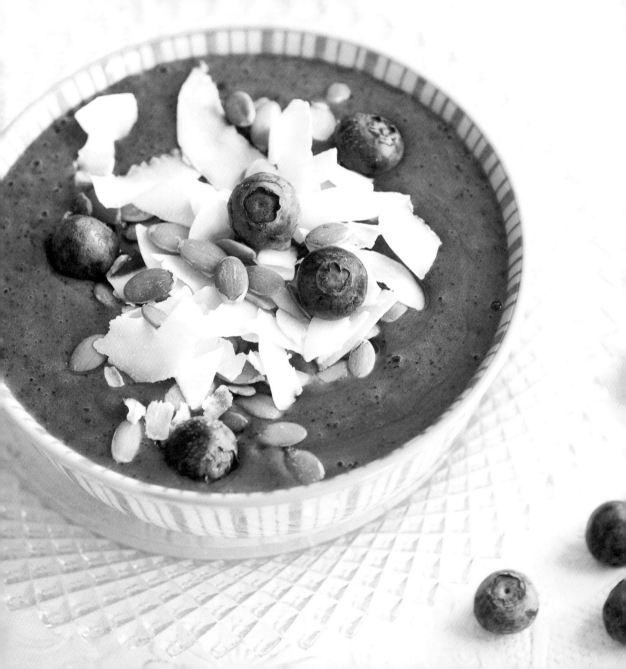

Muscle Max Blueberry Power

This tangy, sweet blend is loaded with protein and complex carbohydrates for workout recovery. The powerful probiotics increase the availability of nutrients from the berries and cocoa nibs.

Serves 2

SMOOTHIE

2 cups blueberries

$1/2$ cup coconut milk yogurt

$1/4$ cup protein powder

$1/4$ cup hulled hemp seeds

1 teaspoon probiotic powder

Combine all the ingredients in a blender and blend until smooth.

TOPPINGS

$1/2$ cup peeled, sliced banana

2 tablespoons unsweetened flaked coconut

2 tablespoons cocoa nibs

Pour the smoothie into two small bowls and sprinkle each with half of the toppings and serve.

NUTRITION FACTS (GRAMS PER SERVING)
Calories 330, Fat 15, Protein 19, Carbs 36, Fiber 8, Net Carbs 28

Probiotic-rich foods and supplements improve digestion and metabolism and enhance the absorption of such nutrients as B vitamins and anthocyanins. Probiotics have also been found to improve inflammatory skin diseases, such as dermatitis, eczema, and psoriasis.

Vanilla Coconut Charger

This hearty, delicately spiced bowl contains stimulating spices for the digestive processes and circulation.

Serves 2

SMOOTHIE

2 bananas, peeled

1 (1-inch) piece turmeric root, peeled and minced

1 cup coconut milk yogurt

¼ cup raisins

¼ cup protein powder

1 tablespoon nut butter

1 tablespoon pure vanilla extract, or 2 vanilla beans (optional)

1 teaspoon ground cinnamon

1 teaspoon probiotic powder

Combine all the ingredients in a blender and blend until smooth.

TOPPINGS

¼ cup peeled, sliced banana

2 tablespoons raisins

2 tablespoons toasted unsweetened flaked coconut

Pinch of salt

Pour the smoothie into two small bowls and sprinkle each with half of the toppings and serve.

NUTRITION FACTS (GRAMS PER SERVING)
Calories 242, Fat 5, Protein 15, Carbs 32, Fiber 4, Net Carbs 28

Nut butters are a rich source of the amino acid leucine, which plays a role in preserving muscle mass during weight loss, raising metabolism, and increasing fat burn.

Power Granola Bowl

Bananas are mood boosters and the omega-3 fatty acids found in the pumpkin seeds help reduce the risk of depression, in this thick and creamy blend.

Serves 2

SMOOTHIE

1 banana, peeled

$1/2$ cup coconut milk yogurt

$1/4$ cup soaked almonds

$1/4$ cup chia seeds

2 tablespoons chopped banana peel

1 teaspoon unsweetened cocoa powder

1 teaspoon ground cinnamon

Combine all the ingredients in a blender and blend until smooth.

TOPPINGS

$1/2$ cup peeled, sliced banana

2 tablespoons toasted unsweetened flaked coconut

2 tablespoons granola

2 tablespoons raisins

Pour the smoothie into two small bowls and sprinkle each with half of the toppings and serve.

NUTRITION FACTS (GRAMS PER SERVING)
Calories 343, Fat 19, Protein 11, Carbs 43, Fiber 16, NetCarbs 27

Bananas are a good source of tryptophan, a precursor to serotonin, a brain chemical that helps regulate mood. The peel is rich in phenolic compounds and flavonoids, which reduce the neurological inflammation that contributes to memory loss and depression.

Strawberry Pecan Power

This comforting combination is packed with
protein for sustained energy and blood sugar regulation.

Serves 2

SMOOTHIE

1 banana, peeled
$1/2$ cup strawberry halves
$1/4$ cup almond milk
$1/4$ cup hulled hemp seeds
$1/4$ cup protein powder
1 teaspoon ground cinnamon

Combine all the ingredients in
a blender and blend until smooth.

TOPPINGS

$1/2$ cup sliced strawberries
$1/2$ cup peeled, sliced banana
2 tablespoons chopped pecans
Pinch of salt

Pour the smoothie into two small
bowls and divide the toppings over
each and serve.

NUTRITION FACTS (GRAMS PER SERVING)
Calories 310, Fat 14, Protein 19, Carb 30, Fiber 7, Net Carbs 23

Protein powder from vegan sources, such as peas, rice, and hemp, contain fiber and provide the amino acids necessary for memory, weight loss, energy, and immune function.

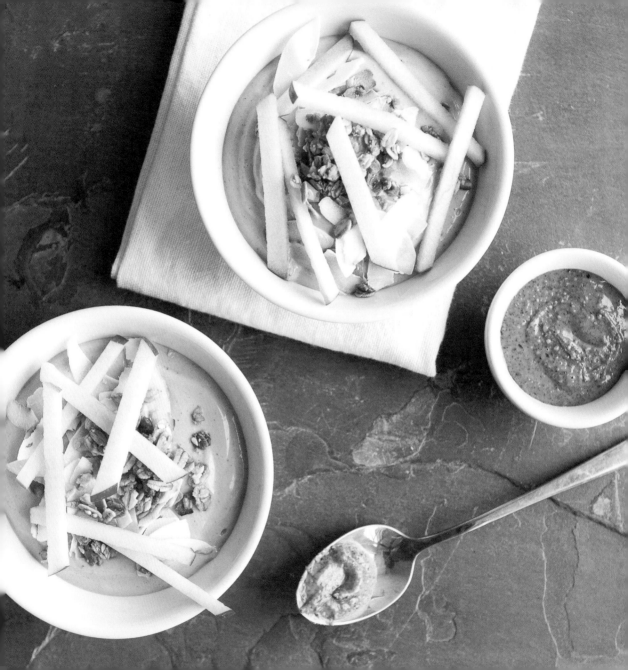

Banana Nut Crunch

This blend has balanced fruit and nut flavors that provide bioactive compounds beneficial to heart health. It is topped with apple with crunchy granola and coconut flakes for flavor and texture.

Serves 2

SMOOTHIE

2 bananas, peeled

$1/4$ cup almond milk

$1/4$ cup hulled hemp seeds

2 tablespoons almond butter

Combine all the ingredients in a blender and blend until smooth.

TOPPINGS

2 tablespoons sliced apple

2 tablespoons granola

2 tablespoons toasted unsweetened flaked coconut

Pour the smoothie into two small bowls and sprinkle each with half of the toppings and serve.

NUTRITION FACTS (GRAMS PER SERVING)
Calories 254, Fat 8, Protein 7, Carbs 40, Fiber 7, NetCarbs 33

Frequent nut consumption has a beneficial effect of lowering the risk of cardiovascular disease as they provide healthy fats and bioactive compounds, such as arginine, fiber, minerals, vitamin E, phytosterols, and polyphenols.

Chocolate Macadamia Pudding

This deliciously thick blend is perfect for a healthy dessert. The omega-3 fatty acids found in macadamia nuts help support brain function.

Serves 2

SMOOTHIE

1 banana, peeled

$1/2$ cup coconut milk yogurt

$1/4$ cup macadamia nuts

$1/4$ cup chia seeds

2 tablespoons unsweetened cocoa powder

2 tablespoons pure vanilla extract

Combine all the ingredients in a blender and blend until smooth.

TOPPINGS

$1/2$ cup peeled, sliced banana

2 tablespoons macadamia nuts

2 tablespoons toasted unsweetened flaked coconut

Pour the smoothie into two small bowls and sprinkle each with half of the toppings and serve.

NUTRITION FACTS (GRAMS PER SERVING)
Calories 319, Fat 22, Protein 8, Carbs 31, Fiber 14, NetCarbs 17

Omega-3 fatty acids found in nuts and seeds, such as pumpkin seeds, walnuts, flaxseeds, and macadamia nuts, reduce the risk for depression.

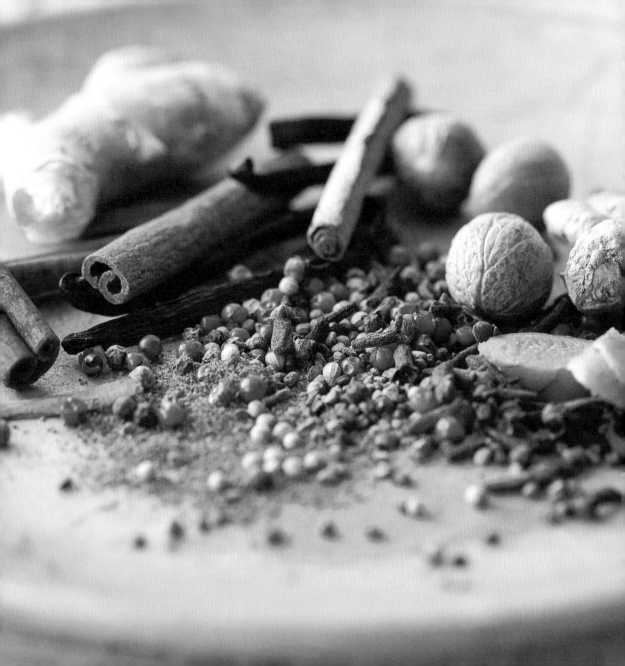

CHAPTER

8

SPICE BOWL RECIPES

Almond Chai

This delicious bowl has powerful spices and zesty lime. Compounds found in turmeric calm inflammation and aid in the prevention of disease.

Serves 2

SMOOTHIE

2 bananas, peeled

1 (1-inch) piece turmeric root, peeled and minced

1/4 lime, chopped with peel (seeds removed)

1/4 cup almond milk

1/4 cup hulled hemp seeds

1 teaspoon ground cardamom

Pinch of ground cloves

Pinch of freshly ground black pepper

Combine all the ingredients in a blender and blend until smooth.

TOPPINGS

2 tablespoons sliced almonds

2 tablespoons cocoa nibs

2 tablespoons hulled hemp seeds

Pour the smoothie into two small bowls and sprinkle each with half of the toppings and serve.

NUTRITION FACTS (GRAMS PER SERVING)
Calories 236, Fat 10, Protein 9, Carbs 30, Fiber 7, NetCarbs 23

Curcumin, a phytochemical found in the root of turmeric, contains anti-inflammatory activity and helps prevent inflammatory conditions, such as ulcerative colitis, rheumatoid arthritis, esophagitis, atherosclerosis, and diabetes.

Creamy Cocoa Crunch

This chocolaty bowl is topped with sliced almonds and cocoa nibs for a satisfying crunch. The cocoa nibs and cocoa powder deliver compounds to help reduce wrinkles and boost the skin's elasticity.

Serves 2

SMOOTHIE

2 bananas, peeled

$1/2$ cup coconut milk yogurt

$1/4$ cup protein powder

$1/4$ cup hulled hemp seeds

2 tablespoons unsweetened cocoa powder

Pinch of salt

Combine all the ingredients in a blender and blend until smooth.

TOPPINGS

2 tablespoons cocoa nibs

2 tablespoons sliced almonds

Pinch of unsweetened cocoa powder

Pour the smoothie into two small bowls and sprinkle each with half of the toppings and serve.

NUTRITION FACTS (GRAMS PER SERVING)
Calories 250, Fat 7, Protein 18, Carbs 27, Fiber 6, NetCarbs 21

A recent study on the benefits of cocoa in improving sun-aged facial skin, wrinkles, and skin elasticity found that just $1/2$ teaspoon of unsweetened cocoa powder per day provides enough cocoa flavonoids to reduce wrinkle depth and discoloration, and improve elasticity. The study's participants experienced these impressive improvements after just a few weeks of daily cocoa ingestion.

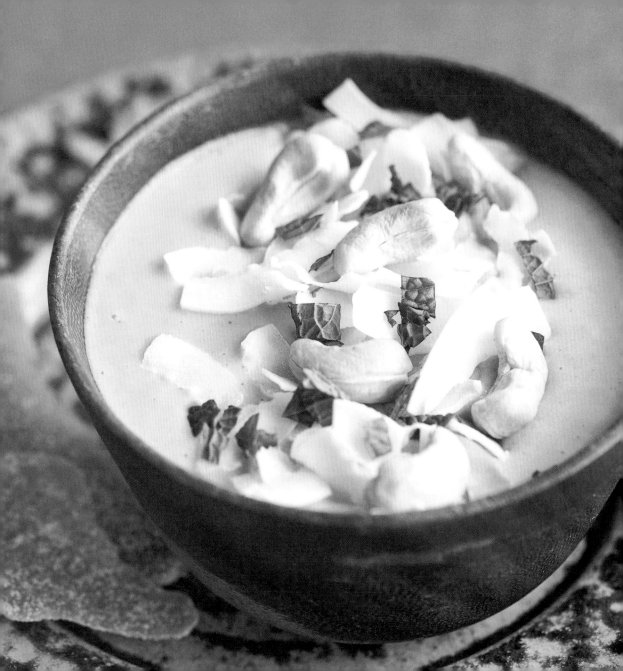

Pineapple Ginger Mango

This delicious bowl blends tropical fruits with fresh turmeric.

Serves 2

SMOOTHIE

1 (1-inch) piece turmeric root, peeled and minced

1 (1-inch) piece ginger root, peeled and minced

1 cup pitted and peeled mango

1 cup chopped pineapple (rind removed)

$1/4$ cup toasted hulled hemp seeds

$1/4$ cup coconut milk beverage

Pinch of freshly ground black pepper

Combine all the ingredients in a blender and blend until smooth.

TOPPINGS

2 tablespoons unsweetened flaked coconut

2 tablespoons cashews

2 teaspoons minced fresh mint leaves

Pour the smoothie into two small bowls and sprinkle each with half of the toppings and serve.

NUTRITION FACTS (GRAMS PER SERVING)
Calories 227, Fat 10, Protein 7, Carbs 29, Fiber 5, NetCarbs 24

Curcumin, the active ingredient in the spice turmeric, is beneficial in the repair of photo-damaged skin, including pigmentary changes, thinning of the skin, and premalignant lesions.

Ginger Snap

This mouthwatering bowl, reminiscent of a freshly baked cookie, contains curcumin from turmeric, eugenol from cloves, piperine from black pepper, and gingerol from ginger, which protect against a range of cancers and diseases.

Serves 4

SMOOTHIE

1 (2-inch) piece ginger root, peeled and minced

2 bananas, peeled

1 (1-inch) piece turmeric root, peeled and minced

1/2 cup soaked almonds

1 cup almond milk

1/4 cup hulled hemp seeds

1 teaspoon ground cinnamon

1/2 teaspoon ground cloves

Combine all the ingredients in a blender and blend until smooth.

TOPPINGS

1/4 cup hulled hemp seeds

1/4 cup sliced almonds

Pinch of ground cinnamon

Pinch of freshly ground black pepper

Pour the smoothie into four small bowls and sprinkle each with one quarter of the toppings and serve.

NUTRITION FACTS (GRAMS PER SERVING)
Calories 310, Fat 22, Protein 12, Carbs 22, Fiber 6, Net Carbs 16

The spices in this blend possess potent antioxidant, anti-inflammatory, antimutagenic, and anticancer activities.

Banana Vanilla Cocoa

This subtly sweet bowl has deep chocolate flavor.

Serves 2

SMOOTHIE

2 bananas, peeled

1 (1-inch) piece turmeric root, peeled and minced

1 (1-inch) piece ginger root, peeled and minced

1 cup hemp milk

$1/4$ cup hulled hemp seeds

$1/4$ cup vanilla protein powder

1 tablespoon unsweetened cocoa powder

1 tablespoon ground cinnamon

1 teaspoon pure vanilla extract

Combine all the ingredients in a blender and blend until smooth.

TOPPINGS

$1/2$ cup peeled, sliced banana

2 tablespoons toasted hulled hemp seeds

2 tablespoons cocoa nibs

1 tablespoon minced candied ginger

Pinch of saffron threads

1 teaspoon ground cardamom

Pinch of freshly ground black pepper

Pour the smoothie into two small bowls and sprinkle each with half of the toppings and serve.

NUTRITION FACTS (GRAMS PER SERVING)
Calories 340, Fat 14, Protein 23, Carbs 36, Fiber 9, Net Carbs 27

A recent study found that after just two months of daily ingestion of cinnamon, cardamom, ginger, and saffron, participants showed significant improvements in total cholesterol, LDL, and HDL levels as well as a reduction in oxidative stress and inflammation.

Vanilla Bean Pot de Crème

This elegant bowl is reminiscent of the classic dessert. This blend contains powerful probiotics for belly health, anti-inflammatory vanilla beans, and added protein to aid in weight management.

Serves 2

SMOOTHIE

2 bananas, peeled

1 cup coconut milk yogurt

$1/4$ cup hulled hemp seeds

$1/4$ cup protein powder

2 teaspoons pure vanilla extract, or two vanilla beans (optional)

Pinch of salt

Combine all the ingredients in a blender and blend until smooth.

TOPPINGS

2 tablespoons chopped strawberries

2 tablespoons toasted almonds

2 tablespoons toasted unsweetened flaked coconut

Pour the smoothie into two small bowls and sprinkle each with half of the toppings and serve.

NUTRITION FACTS (GRAMS PER SERVING)
Calories 272, Fat 9, Protein 18, Carbs 30, Fiber 7, Net Carbs 23

Coconut provides trace minerals, including sodium, magnesium, manganese, and concentrated amounts of potassium, which support neurological function.

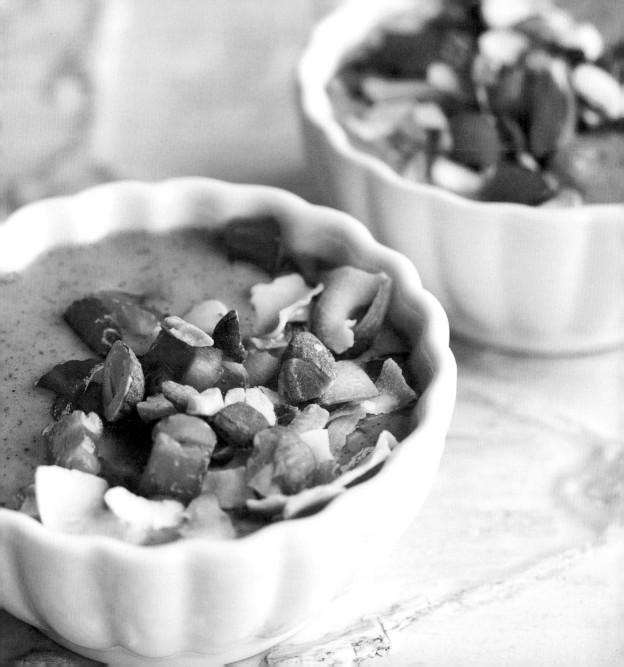

Vanilla Avocado Whip

This nourishing bowl is rich in fatty acids from avocado
and vanillin from vanilla, both of which help keep the skin hydrated,
youthful, and protected from harmful UVB rays.

Serves 2

SMOOTHIE

$^1/_2$ avocado, pitted and peeled

$^1/_2$ cup almond milk

$^1/_4$ cup protein powder

$^1/_4$ cup hulled hemp seeds

2 teaspoons pure vanilla extract,
or 2 vanilla beans (optional)

Combine all the ingredients in a
blender and blend until smooth.

TOPPINGS

$^1/_2$ cup peeled, sliced banana

2 tablespoons toasted hemp seeds

2 tablespoons pumpkin seeds

Pour the smoothie into two small
bowls and sprinkle each with half
of the toppings and serve.

NUTRITION FACTS (GRAMS PER SERVING)
Calories 321, Fat 17, Protein 22, Carbs 18, Fiber 8, NetCarbs 10

Ultraviolet-B (UVB) radiation is a significant factor in the skin aging and skin cancer.
Vanillin, a bioactive compound in vanilla beans, significantly reduces UVB ray damage.

Pumpkin Vanilla Cream

This comforting, spicy blend has crunchy bites
of toasted seeds and is evocative of fresh pumpkin pie.

Serves 4

SMOOTHIE

1 (1-inch) piece ginger root,
peeled and minced

2 cups pure pumpkin purée

$^1/_2$ cup vanilla almond milk

$^1/_4$ cup toasted hulled hemp seeds

$^1/_4$ cup vanilla protein powder

2 teaspoons pure vanilla extract,
or 2 vanilla beans (optional)

Combine all the ingredients in
a blender and blend until smooth.

TOPPINGS

$^1/_4$ cup pumpkin seeds

$^1/_4$ cup toasted sunflower seeds

$^1/_4$ cup toasted hulled hemp seeds

2 teaspoons citrus zest

1 teaspoon freshly grated nutmeg

1 teaspoon ground cinnamon

Pinch of ground cloves

Pour the smoothie into four small
bowls and sprinkle each with one
quarter of the toppings and serve.

NUTRITION FACTS (GRAMS PER SERVING)
Calories 240, Fat 17, Protein 12, Carbs 14, Fiber 7, Net Carbs 7

Cinnamon, cloves, and citrus peel contain oils that provide antibacterial action to help prevent and treat infections. Pumpkin is rich in carotenoids that support vision and weight loss.

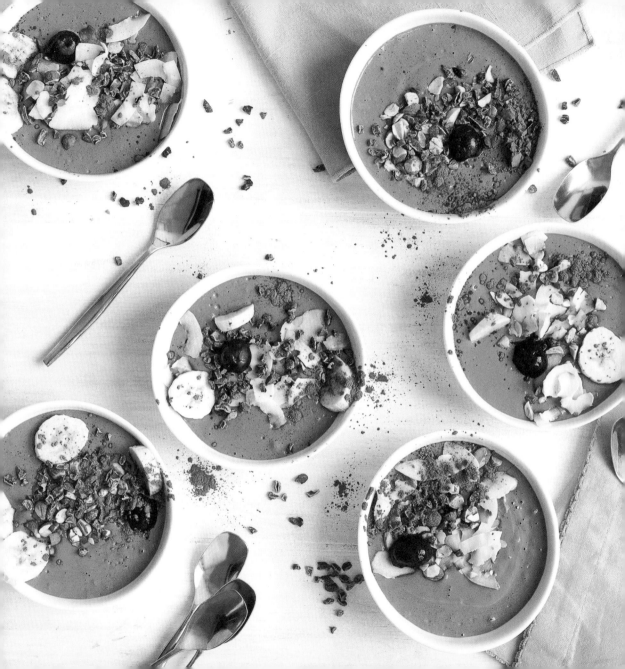

Ice Cream Sundae

A perfect dessert, this simple bowl has intense chocolate
flavor and creamy texture from the coconut milk yogurt.

Serves 2

SMOOTHIE

2 bananas, peeled
$^1/_2$ cup coconut milk yogurt
$^1/_4$ cup hulled hemp seeds
2 tablespoons unsweetened cocoa powder
2 teaspoons pure vanilla extract
2 tablespoons chia seed

Combine all the ingredients in
a blender and blend until smooth.

TOPPINGS

$^1/_2$ cup pitted dark sweet cherries
$^1/_2$ cup peeled, sliced banana
2 tablespoons cocoa nibs
2 tablespoons toasted crushed almonds
2 teaspoons unsweetened cocoa powder
2 tablespoons toasted coconut flakes

Pour the smoothie into two small
bowls and sprinkle each with half
of the toppings and serve.

NUTRITION FACTS (GRAMS PER SERVING)
Calories 373, Fat 16, Protein 14, Carbs 47, Fiber 18, NetCarbs 29

Melatonin from banana and its peel contributes to quality of sleep and weight loss.
Bananas are an excellent source of potassium and vitamin B_6, which protect against
insomnia and irritability. They also provide fructooligosaccharide, which encourages the
growth of healthy bacteria in the digestive system and pectin, which supports digestion.

Cocoa Mood Booster

This bowl has spiced chocolate flavors that are sure to delight.
The coconut milk yogurt provides gut-soothing probiotics,
and fiber helps satiate the appetite for hours.

Serves 2

SMOOTHIE

2 bananas, peeled

1/2 cup coconut milk yogurt

2 tablespoons protein powder

2 tablespoons unsweetened
cocoa powder

1 teaspoon pure vanilla extract

1/4 teaspoon ground cinnamon

Combine all the ingredients in
a blender and blend until smooth.

TOPPINGS

2 tablespoons toasted unsweetened
flaked coconut

2 tablespoons cocoa nibs

2 tablespoons toasted hulled
hemp seeds

1/4 teaspoon freshly grated nutmeg

Pour the smoothie into two small
bowls and sprinkle each with half
of the toppings and serve.

NUTRITION FACTS (GRAMS PER SERVING)
Calories 260, Fat 10, Protein 13, Carbs 37 Fiber 9, NetCarbs 28

Coconut milk yogurt and probiotic supplements provide considerable amounts of healthful microbes that have proven to affect depression. In as little as eight weeks, probiotic supplementation in patients with major depressive disorders showed beneficial effects on depression, insulin, inflammation, and detoxification.

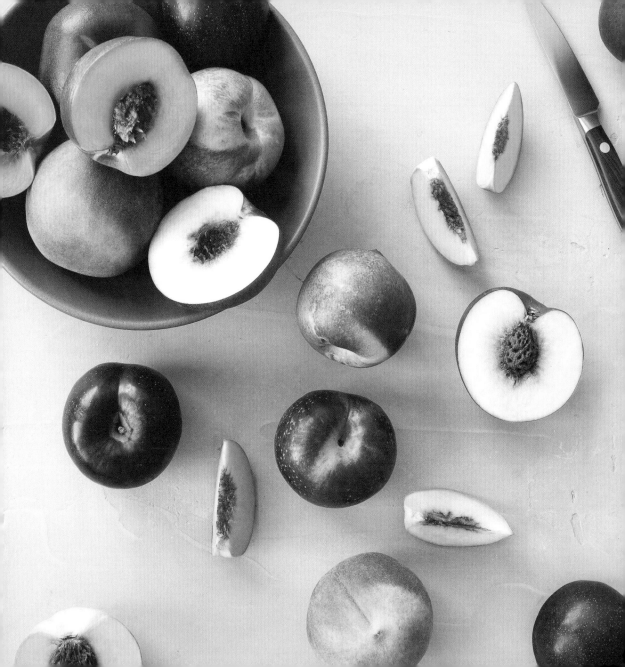

STONE FRUIT BOWL RECIPES

Cinnamon Hazelnut Cream

This nutty, sweet blend has fresh plums and hazelnuts.
The polyphenols in cinnamon help lower cholesterol and reduce weight gain.

Serves 4

SMOOTHIE

2 plums, halved and pitted
1 banana, peeled
$1/2$ cup soaked hazelnuts
$1/2$ cup hemp milk
$1/4$ cup hulled hemp seeds
1 tablespoon pure vanilla extract

Combine all the ingredients in a blender and blend until smooth.

TOPPINGS

1 plum, halved and pitted
1 cup peeled, sliced banana
2 tablespoons chopped hazelnuts
1 teaspoon ground cinnamon

Pour the smoothie into four small bowls and sprinkle each with one quarter of the toppings and serve.

NUTRITION FACTS (GRAMS PER SERVING)
Calories 204, Fat 12, Protein 7, Carbs 20, Fiber 5, NetCarbs 20

Cinnamon polyphenols have been found to repair pancreatic beta cells in initial studies and have also been found to improve lipid profiles and lower cholesterol levels.

Vanilla Cherry Banana

This delicious and melatonin-rich bowl is sure to lull you into a restful slumber.

Serves 2

SMOOTHIE

1 banana, peeled

2 cups pitted dark sweet cherries

$^1/_4$ cup hulled hemp seeds

$^1/_4$ cup protein powder

3 tablespoons black cherry juice concentrate

2 tablespoons pure vanilla extract, or 2 vanilla beans (optional)

2 tablespoons chopped banana peel

Combine all the ingredients in a blender and blend until smooth.

TOPPINGS

$^1/_2$ cup peeled, sliced banana

$^1/_2$ cup cherry halves

2 tablespoons hulled hemp seeds

Pour the smoothie into two small bowls and sprinkle each with half of the toppings and serve.

NUTRITION FACTS (GRAMS PER SERVING)
Calories 380, Fat 18, Protein 25, Carbs 37 Fiber 10, NetCarbs 27

This bowl contains concentrated amounts of melatonin from cherries, cherry juice, banana, and banana skin that support deep, restful sleep.

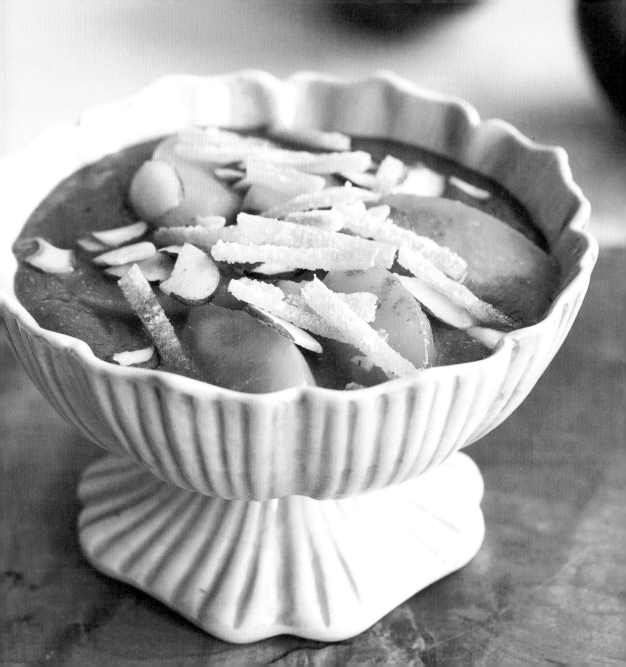

Summer Peaches and Ginger

This combination is spicy and sweet with fresh ginger root that soothes the stomach. Apricot, peaches, and cherries are off the charts in antioxidant polyphenols, which provide protection from the development of type 2 diabetes mellitus.

Serves 4

SMOOTHIE

1 peach, halved and pitted

1 (1-inch) piece ginger root, peeled and minced

1 (1-inch) piece turmeric root, peeled and minced

1 apricot, halved and pitted

1/2 cup pitted dark sweet cherries

1/2 cup almond milk

1/4 cup chia seeds

Combine all the ingredients in a blender and blend until smooth.

TOPPINGS

1/4 cup sliced peach

2 tablespoons sliced almonds

1 tablespoon chopped candied ginger

1 teaspoon ground cinnamon

1/2 teaspoon freshly grated nutmeg

Pinch of freshly ground black pepper

Pour the smoothie into four small bowls and sprinkle each with one quarter of the toppings and serve.

NUTRITION FACTS (GRAMS PER SERVING)
Calories 105, Fat 5, Protein 4, Carbs 22, Fiber 7, NetCarbs 15

Stone fruit polyphenols modulate insulin secretion in pancreatic cells and target insulin-sensitive tissues to enhance glucose transport.

Almond Cardamom Peach

This gorgeous bowl has sweet fruits and aromatic spices.
Peaches contain powerful compounds that sharpen the mind.

Serves 2

SMOOTHIE

1 cup sliced peach

1 (1-inch) piece turmeric root,
peeled and minced

1/2 cup pitted dark sweet cherries

1/2 cup almond milk

Combine all the ingredients in a blender and blend until smooth.

TOPPINGS

1/2 cup chopped peach

1/2 cup cherry halves

2 tablespoons sliced almonds

1 teaspoon ground cardamom

1 teaspoon ground cinnamon

Pour the smoothie into two small bowls and sprinkle each with half of the toppings and serve.

NUTRITION FACTS (GRAMS PER SERVING)
Calories 130, Fat 5, Protein 4, Carbs 21, Fiber 4, NetCarbs 17

Peaches are rich in carotenoids, including lutein and zeaxanthin, which support vision, memory, and cognitive performance in the young and elderly.

Cinnamon Peach

Fresh fruit blends beautifully with soaked almonds in this bowl.
The essential vitamins provided help reduce wrinkles, calm
inflammation, and enhance the skin's elasticity and texture.

Serves 2

SMOOTHIE

1 nectarine, pitted

$1/2$ cup sliced peach

$1/2$ cup pitted dark sweet cherries

$1/2$ cup hemp milk

$1/4$ cup soaked almonds

$1/4$ cup hulled hemp seeds

Combine all the ingredients in
a blender and blend until smooth.

TOPPINGS

$1/2$ cup cherry halves

2 tablespoons hulled hemp seeds

Pinch of ground cinnamon

Pour the smoothie into two small
bowls and sprinkle each with half
of the toppings and serve.

NUTRITION FACTS (GRAMS PER SERVING)
Calories 390, Fat 25, Protein 16, Carbs 31, Fiber 7, Net Carbs 24

The polyphenols from the stone fruit, as well as the vitamin B_3, vitamin C, and vitamin E
in this bowl improve skin texture and firmness.

Cherry Lemonade

This blend is an immune-boosting treat. Cherries and zesty lemon provide powerful antioxidants and are both sources of vitamin C.

Serves 2

SMOOTHIE

1 banana, peeled

$^1/_4$ lemon with peel, chopped (seeds removed)

2 cups pitted dark sweet cherries

$^1/_4$ cup chia seeds

3 tablespoons cherry juice concentrate

Combine all the ingredients in a blender and blend until smooth.

TOPPINGS

$^1/_2$ cup pitted dark sweet cherries

2 tablespoons lemon zest

2 tablespoons hulled hemp seeds

2 tablespoons sliced almonds

Pour the smoothie into two small bowls and sprinkle each with half of the toppings and serve.

NUTRITION FACTS (GRAMS PER SERVING)
Calories 200, Fat 8, Protein 6, Carbs 29, Fiber 4, Net Carbs 25

The immune system is extremely vulnerable to dietary oxidants (such as sugar) and environmental oxidants (such as air pollution and household chemicals) as uncontrolled free radicals impair its function and defense mechanisms. Cherries and cherry juice provide active antioxidant compounds, including phenolics and anthocyanins, which disarm free radicals, rendering them harmless.

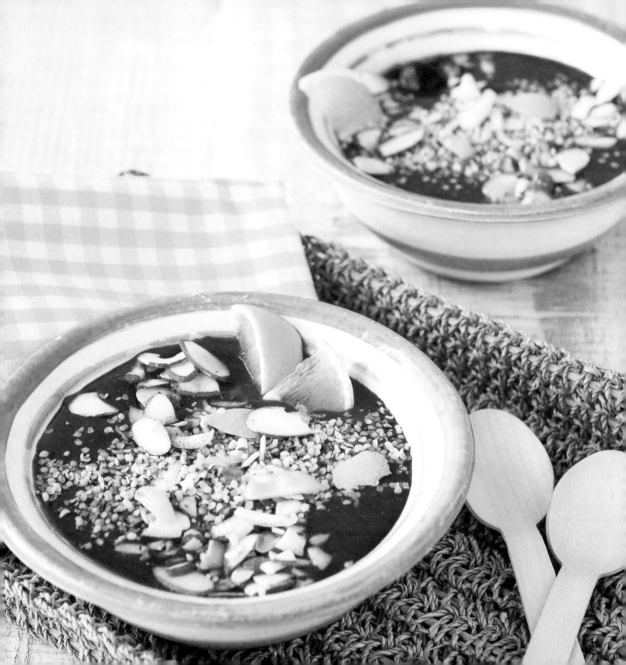

Cashew Cherry Crunch

This bowl is a balanced blend of greens, fruits, nuts, and seeds.

Serves 4

SMOOTHIE

1 cup sliced peach

1 cup fresh spinach leaves

1 cup almond milk

$1/2$ cup soaked almonds

$1/2$ cup cashews

$1/4$ cup toasted hulled hemp seeds

$1/4$ cup protein powder

Combine all the ingredients in a blender and blend until smooth.

TOPPINGS

$1/2$ cup chopped peach

$1/2$ cup chopped apricot

$1/2$ cup cherry halves

Pour the smoothie into four small bowls and sprinkle each with one quarter of the toppings and serve.

NUTRITION FACTS (GRAMS PER SERVING)
Calories 310, Fat 20, Protein 16, Carbs 22, Fiber 5, Net Carbs 17

Nuts and seeds are rich sources of alpha-lipoic acid and chromium that support blood sugar regulation and diabetes management, providing protection against hypo- and hyperglycemia.

Apricot Nutmeg Granola

This bowl is sweet, spicy, and rich in fiber. Nutmeg contributes powerful antibacterial properties and turmeric quells inflammation.

Serves 2

SMOOTHIE	TOPPINGS
3 apricots, halved and pitted	2 tablespoons granola
1 (1-inch) piece turmeric root, peeled and minced	2 tablespoons sliced almonds
$^1/_2$ cup almond milk	Pinch of ground cinnamon
$^1/_4$ cup hulled hemp seeds	1 teaspoon ground cinnamon
1 teaspoon pure vanilla extract	$^1/_4$ teaspoon freshly grated nutmeg
	Pinch of freshly ground black pepper

Combine all the ingredients in a blender and blend until smooth.

Pour the smoothie into two small bowls and sprinkle each with half of the toppings and serve.

NUTRITION FACTS (GRAMS PER SERVING)
Calories 230, Fat 12, Protein 10, Carbs 21, Fiber 4, Net Carbs 17

Colorectal cancer is the third most common type of cancer in men and women in the United States. Nutmeg, which exhibits antimicrobial activity, helps protect the colon from cancer development through its anti-inflammatory action, modulation of gut microbiota, and by improving lipid metabolism.

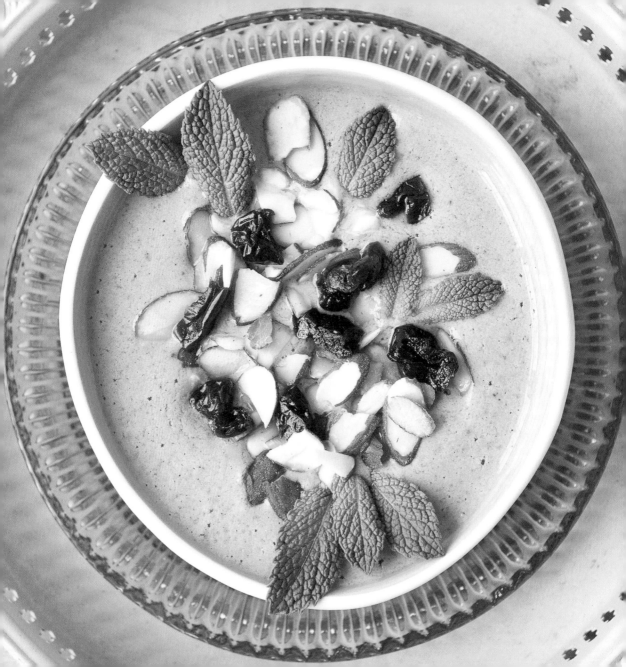

Creamy Strawberry Mint

This tangy, sweet bowl has added protein to help
suppress appetite and provide important amino acids.

Serves 2

SMOOTHIE

1 cup pitted dark sweet cherries

1 cup strawberry halves

$1/2$ cup coconut milk yogurt

$1/4$ cup hulled hemp seeds

$1/4$ cup protein powder

1 teaspoon probiotic powder

Combine all the ingredients in
a blender and blend until smooth.

TOPPINGS

2 tablespoons chopped dried cherries

2 tablespoons sliced almonds

Sprigs of fresh mint leaves

Pour the smoothie into two small
bowls and sprinkle each with half
of the toppings and serve.

NUTRITION FACTS (GRAMS PER SERVING)
Calories 260, Fat 13, Protein 19, Carbs 21, Fiber 5, Net Carbs 16

Supplementation of probiotics and dietary intake of prebiotics via plant foods, such as
berries, can induce favorable changes in the gut bacterial species and improve blood
sugar balance. This is critical for those with hypoglycemia and diabetes.

Cherry Cocoa Crunch

This balanced blend has spiced fragrance and sweet fruits. Cherries contain high levels of molecules involved in mood regulation and stress reduction.

Serves 2

SMOOTHIE

1 banana, peeled

1 (1-inch) piece turmeric root, peeled and minced

1 cup pitted dark sweet cherries

1 cup fresh spinach leaves

1/2 cup carrot juice

1/4 cup hulled hemp seeds

Combine all the ingredients in a blender and blend until smooth.

TOPPINGS

1/2 cup peeled, sliced banana

2 tablespoons cocoa nibs

2 tablespoons toasted hulled hemp seeds

2 tablespoons unsweetened cocoa powder

Pinch of freshly ground black pepper

Pour the smoothie into two small bowls and sprinkle each with half of the toppings and serve.

NUTRITION FACTS (GRAMS PER SERVING)
Calories 280, Fat 15, Protein 13, Carbs 30, Fiber 9, Net Carbs 21

Cherries contain high levels of tryptophan, serotonin, and melatonin that help reduce the level of stress hormones, such as cortisol, in the blood.

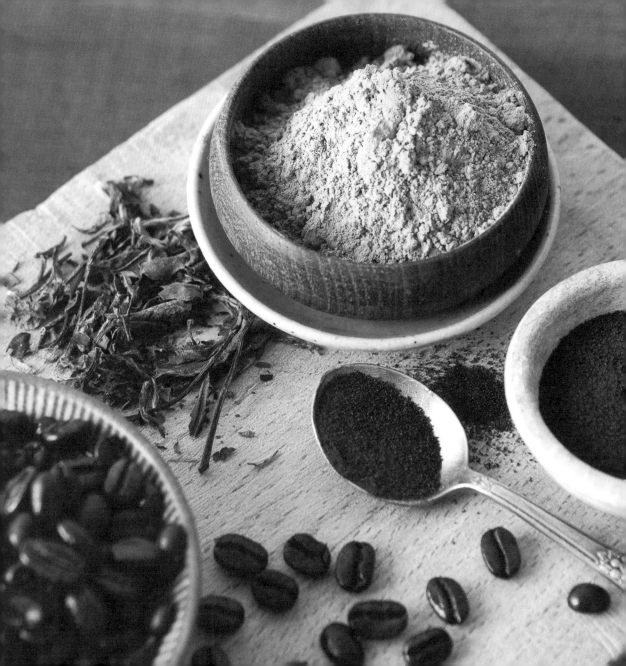

TEA & COFFEE
BOWL
RECIPES

Cherry Matcha

Deep red in color, this bowl has sweet and complex notes. Matcha powder adds compounds that support weight loss and reduce the risk of many chronic diseases.

Serves 2

SMOOTHIE

1 banana, peeled

2 cups pitted dark sweet cherries

$^1/_2$ cup black currant juice

$^1/_4$ cup chia seeds

1 tablespoon matcha powder

1 teaspoon pure vanilla extract

Combine all the ingredients in a blender and blend until smooth.

TOPPINGS

$^1/_2$ cup cherry halves

$^1/_2$ cup sliced kumquat

$^1/_2$ cup peeled, sliced banana

Pour the smoothie into two small bowls and sprinkle each with half of the toppings and serve.

NUTRITION FACTS (GRAMS PER SERVING)
Calories 300, Fat 11, Protein 8, Carbs 49, Fiber 17, Net Carbs 32

Green tea polyphenols are abundant in tea leaves and even more concentrated in matcha powder (ground tea leaves). Regular consumption of green tea has been associated with a reduced risk of cancer and of cardiovascular and neurodegenerative diseases.

Pineapple Matcha Refresher

This powerful anti-inflammatory bowl is rich in tropical pineapple and coconut flavors with fragrant and juicy toppings.

Serves 2

SMOOTHIE

1 cup orange segments

1 (1-inch piece) turmeric root, peeled and minced

1 cup chopped pineapple (rind removed)

1/2 cup coconut milk beverage

1/4 cup chia seeds

1 tablespoon matcha powder

Combine all the ingredients in a blender and blend until smooth.

TOPPINGS

1/2 cup orange segments

1/2 cup chopped walnuts

Pinch of matcha powder

Pinch of freshly ground black pepper

Pour the smoothie into two small bowls and sprinkle each with half of the toppings and serve.

NUTRITION FACTS (GRAMS PER SERVING)
Calories 240, Fat 10, Protein 7, Carbs 36, Fiber 14, Net Carbs 22

Walnuts are a rich source of anti-inflammatory alpha-linoleic acid, which provides protection of the urologic organs (bladder, kidney, and prostate) and associated conditions, such as bladder pain syndrome, bladder cancer, prostate cancer, and chronic pelvic pain syndrome, by suppressing urologic inflammation.

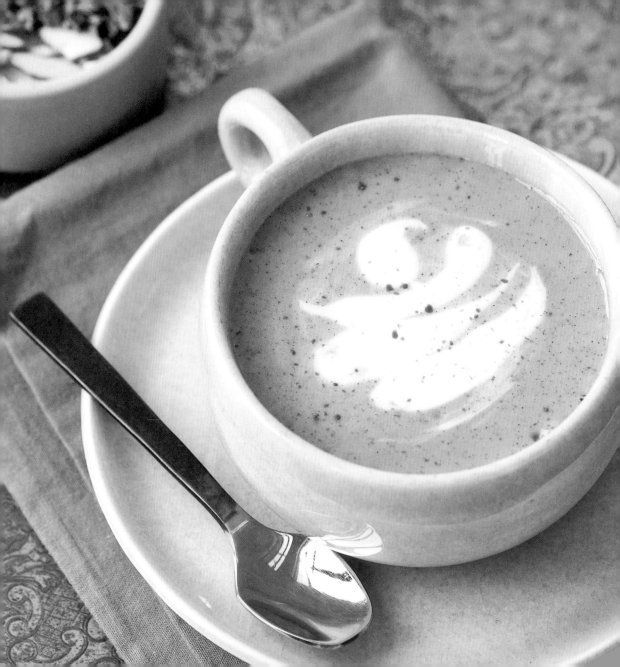

Almond Matcha Latte

This bowl is has an exotic, earthy, umami flavor. The Japanese culinary term *umami* means "savory" or "delicious," and describes matcha well.

Serves 2

SMOOTHIE

2 bananas, peeled

1/2 cup coconut milk yogurt

1/4 cup hulled hemp seeds

1/4 cup vanilla protein powder

1 tablespoon matcha powder

1 tablespoon pure vanilla extract

Combine all the ingredients in a blender and blend until smooth.

TOPPINGS

2 tablespoons sliced almonds

2 tablespoons cocoa nibs

2 tablespoons coconut milk yogurt

Pinch of matcha powder

Pour the smoothie into two small bowls and sprinkle each with half of the toppings and serve.

NUTRITION FACTS (GRAMS PER SERVING)
Calories 314, Fat 13, Protein 20, Carbs 30, Fiber 7, Net Carbs 23

Matcha powder is a rich source of policosanol, which provides cardiovascular protection by inhibiting cholesterol production.

Caffè Borgia

This delicate orange flavored bowl has a light espresso
base with juicy tangerine and crunchy chocolate toppings.

Serves 2

SMOOTHIE

2 bananas, peeled
1 cup orange segments
$1/4$ cup hemp milk
$1/4$ cup hulled hemp seeds
1 tablespoon instant espresso powder
1 teaspoon pure vanilla extract

Combine all the ingredients in
a blender and blend until smooth.

TOPPINGS

$1/2$ cup tangerine segments
2 tablespoons cocoa nibs
2 tablespoons toasted hulled hemp seeds
2 twists of orange peel

Pour the smoothie into two small
bowls and sprinkle each with half
of the toppings and serve.

NUTRITION FACTS (GRAMS PER SERVING)
Calories 320, Fat 15, Protein 13, Carbs 41, Fiber 8, Net Carbs 33

Coffee intake increases blood levels of the antioxidant caffeic acid, providing protection
from the oxidative stress that causes disease and depression. Its antioxidants support
blood sugar regulation, immune function, and cancer prevention.

Coconut Vanilla Café

In Vietnam, cà phê sua chua (*ca-fe su-aw chu-ah*) or yogurt coffee, is served as a refreshing drink to energize and suppress appetite. This blend is similar as it has rich coffee flavor and tangy, probiotic-rich, coconut milk yogurt.

Serves 2

SMOOTHIE

2 bananas, peeled

1/2 cup coconut milk yogurt

1/4 cup hulled hemp seeds

1 tablespoon pure vanilla extract

1 tablespoon instant espresso powder

Combine all the ingredients in a blender and blend until smooth.

TOPPINGS

1/2 cup peeled, sliced banana

2 tablespoons sliced almonds

2 tablespoons cocoa nibs

Pour the smoothie into two small bowls and sprinkle each with half of the toppings and serve.

NUTRITION FACTS (GRAMS PER SERVING)
Calories 290, Fat 14, Protein 10, Carbs 36, Fiber 8, Net Carbs 28

Coffee contains antioxidants that promote the reduction of water weight and mannoo-ligosaccharides that have been found to reduce body fat in men, when ingested on a consistent basis.

Macchiato Magic

This blend has deep espresso flavor that combines with fiber-rich bananas in a tangy base, and is topped with a dollop of coconut milk yogurt for sustained energy. Ferulic acid, found in coffee, has been shown to fight free radicals.

Serves 4

SMOOTHIE

2 bananas, peeled
$1/2$ cup coconut milk yogurt
$1/4$ cup hulled hemp seeds
2 tablespoons pure vanilla extract
2 tablespoons instant espresso powder

Combine all the ingredients in a blender and blend until smooth.

TOPPINGS

$1/4$ cup coconut milk yogurt
4 wafer cookies

Pour the smoothie into four wide-mouthed cups and dollop the top of each with one quarter of the coconut milk yogurt. Serve the wafer cookies on the side.

NUTRITION FACTS (GRAMS PER SERVING)
Calories 170, Fat 10, Protein 5, Carbs 19, Fiber 3 NetCarbs 16

Coffee is a rich source of the polyphenol antioxidant ferulic acid, which modulates phosphodiesterase, and is involved in the pathogenesis of Alzheimer's disease. Researchers believe this could be the reason that coffee intake appears to reduce the risk for development of Alzheimer's.

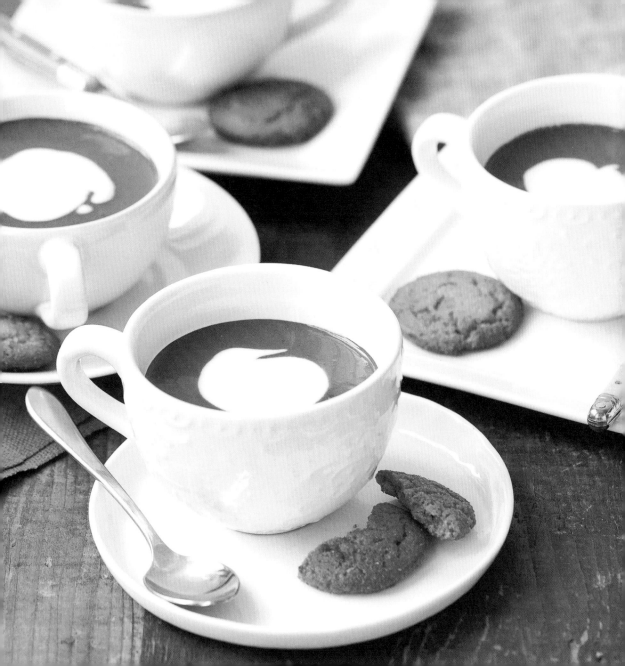

Creamy Matcha Crunch

This sweet, creamy bowl has essential fatty acids and antioxidants to ward off disease and increase cognitive function.

Serves 2

SMOOTHIE

1/2 avocado, pitted and peeled

2 cups red grapes

1/4 cup chia seeds

3 tablespoons black cherry juice concentrate

1 tablespoon matcha powder

Combine all the ingredients in a blender and blend until smooth.

TOPPINGS

2 tablespoons pumpkin seeds

2 tablespoons toasted sliced almonds

2 tablespoons hulled hemp seeds

Pinch of matcha powder

Pour the smoothie into two small bowls and sprinkle each with half of the toppings and serve.

NUTRITION FACTS (GRAMS PER SERVING)
Calories 240, Fat 14, Protein 8, Carbs 25, Fiber 9, NetCarbs 16

Polyphenols are functional compounds in green tea that have the ability to prevent and heal the damage caused by high blood sugar levels, as in the case of diabetic neuropathy and retinopathy.

Chai Coffee

Comforting vanilla blends with espresso and spicy nutmeg in this nutritious bowl. Nutmeg has been shown to relieve pain and calm indigestion.

Serves 2

SMOOTHIE

1 banana, peeled

$^1/_2$ cup hemp milk

$^1/_2$ cup soaked almonds

$^1/_2$ cup hulled hemp seeds

$^1/_4$ cup vanilla protein powder

1 tablespoon instant espresso powder

1 tablespoon pure vanilla extract, or 2 vanilla beans (optional)

1 teaspoon freshly grated nutmeg

Combine all the ingredients in a blender and blend until smooth.

TOPPINGS

$^1/_2$ cup peeled, sliced banana

2 tablespoons toasted almonds

Pinch of freshly grated nutmeg

Pour the smoothie into two small bowls and sprinkle each with half of the toppings and serve.

NUTRITION FACTS (GRAMS PER SERVING)
Calories 310, Fat 21, Protein 18, Carbs 19 Fiber 7, NetCarbs 12

Nutmeg's bioactive components, such as neolignans, phenylpropanoids, phenolics, and triterpenoids, provide antioxidant and anti-inflammatory benefits.

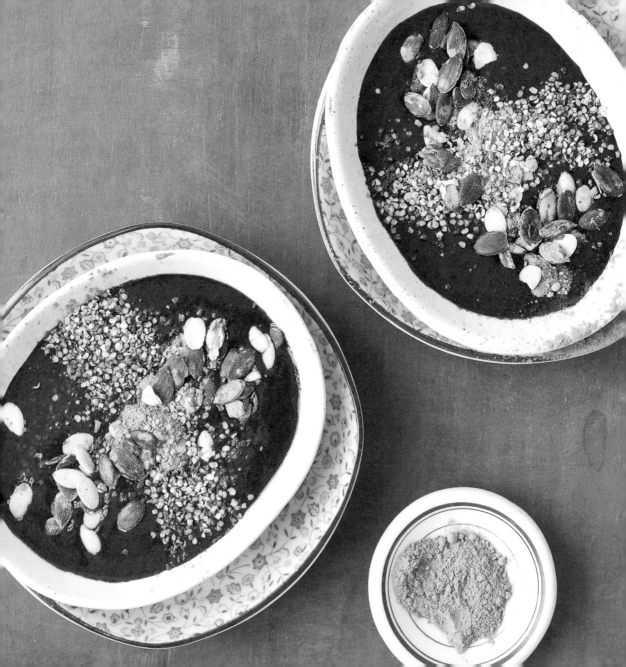

Matcha Blueberry Energizer

This blend contains antioxidant-rich blueberries and powerful polyphenols from green tea to help inhibit premature aging.

Serves 2

SMOOTHIE

1/4 lemon, chopped with peel (seeds removed)

2 cups blueberries

1/2 cup coconut milk beverage

1/4 cup hulled hemp seeds

1 tablespoon matcha powder

Combine all the ingredients in a blender and blend until smooth.

TOPPINGS

2 tablespoons pumpkin seeds

2 tablespoons toasted hulled hemp seeds

Pinch of matcha powder

Pour the smoothie into two small bowls and sprinkle each with half of the toppings and serve.

NUTRITION FACTS (GRAMS PER SERVING)
Calories 310, Fat 20, Protein 13, Carbs 28 Fiber 6, NetCarbs 22

Green tea contains epigallocatechin gallate (EGCG), which supports weight loss, regulates blood sugar, protects against cancer, and supports hair growth by reducing the oxidative stress associated with alopecia.

Power Mocha

This bowl is rich in fiber from banana and hemp seeds, and provides added protein to help control weight gain.

Serves 2

SMOOTHIE

2 bananas, peeled

$1/2$ cup almond milk

$1/4$ cup hulled hemp seeds

$1/4$ cup vanilla protein powder

1 teaspoon pure vanilla extract, or 2 vanilla beans (optional)

2 tablespoons unsweetened cocoa powder

1 tablespoon instant espresso powder

Combine all the ingredients in a blender and blend until smooth.

TOPPINGS

$1/2$ cup peeled, sliced banana

3 tablespoons cocoa nibs

Pinch of ground cinnamon

Pour the smoothie into two small bowls and sprinkle each with half of the toppings and serve.

NUTRITION FACTS (GRAMS PER SERVING)
Calories 380, Fat 16, Protein 24, Carbs 46 Fiber 14, NetCarbs 22

Cocoa and coffee contain large amounts of polyphenols that support energy metabolism and adiposity and obesity. They stimulate lipid metabolism, which helps move fat out of fat cells.

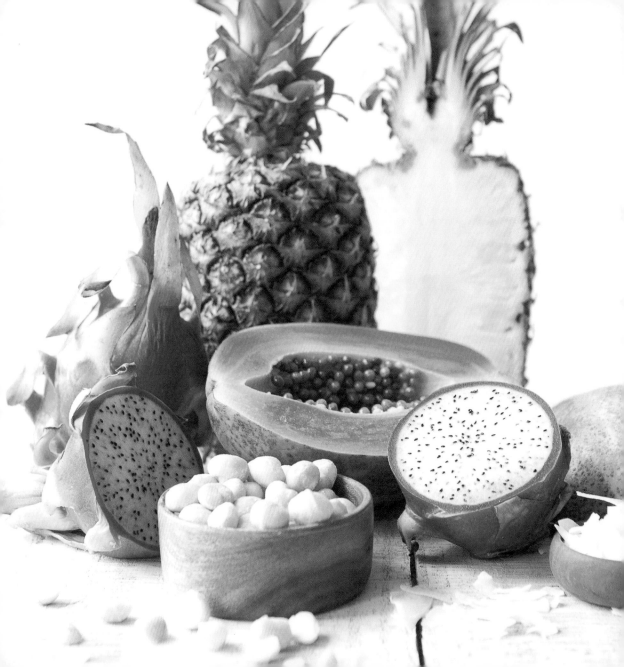

TROPICAL FRUIT BOWL RECIPES

Super Star Fruit

This subtly sweet bowl packs in the medicinal
nutrients that provide antioxidant and antimicrobial effects.

Serves 2

SMOOTHIE

1 banana, peeled

1 (1-inch) piece turmeric root,
peeled and minced

$^1/_2$ cup chopped star fruit

$^1/_2$ cup almond milk

$^1/_4$ cup hulled hemp seeds

Pinch of freshly ground black pepper

Combine all the ingredients in
a blender and blend until smooth.

TOPPINGS

$^1/_2$ cup sliced star fruit

$^1/_2$ cup peeled, sliced banana

2 tablespoons unsweetened
flaked coconut

2 tablespoons toasted sliced almonds

Pour the smoothie into two small
bowls and sprinkle each with half
of the toppings and serve.

NUTRITION FACTS (GRAMS PER SERVING)
Calories 280, Fat 16, Protein 11, Carbs 25, Fiber 6, Net Carbs 19

Carambola, also known as star fruit, provides antioxidants, potassium, vitamin C, and
antimicrobial polyphenolic compounds.

Creamy Coconut Macadamia

This delicious blend is silky from avocado
and filling from fiber-rich macadamia nuts.

Serves 2

SMOOTHIE

1 (1-inch) piece turmeric root,
peeled and minced

1 banana, peeled

1/2 avocado, pitted and peeled

1/2 cup mango nectar

1/4 cup soaked macadamia nuts

1 teaspoon pure vanilla extract

Pinch of freshly ground black pepper

Combine all the ingredients in
a blender and blend until smooth.

TOPPINGS

2 tablespoons chopped
macadamia nuts

2 tablespoons unsweetened
flaked coconut

2 tablespoons pomegranate arils

Pour the smoothie into two small
bowls and sprinkle each with half
of the toppings and serve.

NUTRITION FACTS (GRAMS PER SERVING)
Calories 270, Fat 19, Protein 3, Carbs 27 Fiber 5, NetCarbs 22

Macadamia nuts are rich in phytochemicals, such as phenols, proanthocyanidins, gallic
acid, ellagic acid, and flavonoids, which act as antioxidants that support cognitive function and disease prevention.

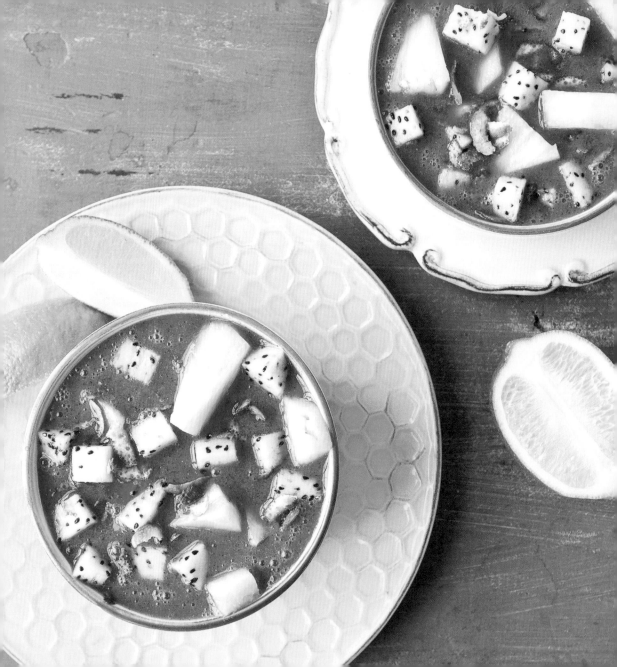

Island Bliss

This beautiful, bright bowl contains exceptionally high antioxidant levels due to its dragon fruit and fresh turmeric root.

Serves 2

SMOOTHIE

1 (1-inch) piece turmeric root, peeled and minced

1/4 lime, chopped with peel (seeds removed)

1 cup chopped dragon fruit (rind removed)

1/2 cup chopped pineapple (rind removed)

1/2 cup coconut milk beverage

1/4 cup hulled hemp seeds

Combine all the ingredients in a blender and blend until smooth.

TOPPINGS

1/4 cup chopped dragon fruit (rind removed)

1/4 cup chopped pineapple (rind removed)

2 tablespoons toasted unsweetened flaked coconut

2 tablespoons lime zest

Pinch of freshly ground black pepper

Pour the smoothie into two small bowls and sprinkle each with half of the toppings and serve.

NUTRITION FACTS (GRAMS PER SERVING)
Calories 220, Fat 12, Protein 8, Carbs 23 Fiber 2, NetCarbs 21

Both red and white dragon fruit, which is also known as pitaya, contain off-the-chart levels of antioxidants, such as phenolics, flavonoids, and ascorbic acid. They are also rich in dietary fiber, ellagic acid, and flavone glycosides. Pitaya phytochemicals improve obesity-related metabolic disorders, such as insulin resistance and fatty liver.

Papaya Lime Macadamia

Fresh island flavors and bright lime come together in this nutritious bowl. High in lycopene, papaya supports the heart and protects the eyes.

Serves 2

SMOOTHIE

¹/₄ lime, chopped with peel (seeds removed)

¹/₂ avocado, pitted and peeled

2 cups peeled papaya

¹/₂ cup coconut milk beverage

¹/₄ cup hulled hemp seeds

Combine all the ingredients in a blender and blend until smooth.

TOPPINGS

¹/₄ cup peeled papaya

2 tablespoons unsweetened flaked coconut

2 tablespoons chopped macadamia nuts

2 tablespoons chopped pistachios

1 teaspoon lime zest

Pour the smoothie into two small bowls and sprinkle each with half of the toppings and serve.

NUTRITION FACTS (GRAMS PER SERVING)
Calories 301, Fat 18, Protein 9, Carbs 28, Fiber 7, Net Carbs 22

Papaya's lycopene increases serum lycopene levels, which not only reduces the risk for developing cardiovascular disease, diabetes, and cancer but also improves the outcome for those with these conditions. Papaya is also a rich source of xanthophyll, which has a protective effect against cataracts and retinopathy.

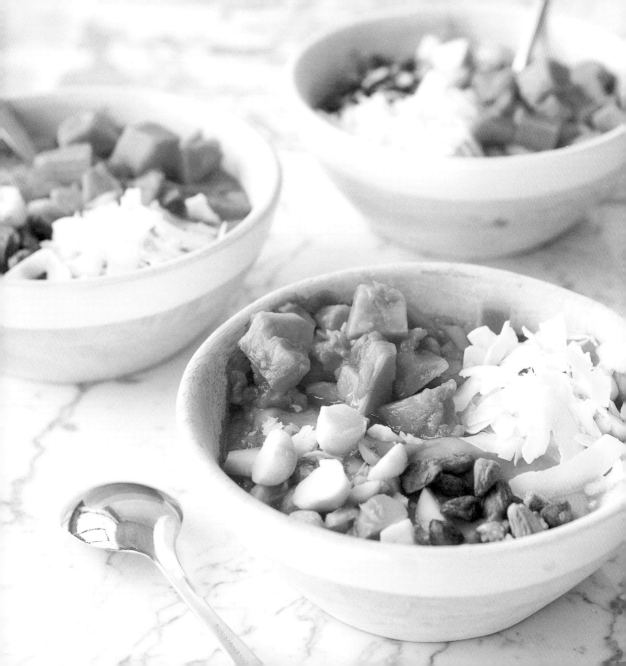

Kiwi Cooler

This light blend has refreshing cucumber and citrus flavor
with crunchy almonds, coconut bites, and fresh mint fragrance.

Serves 2

SMOOTHIE

2 kiwis, peeled

$1/2$ lime with peel, chopped
(seeds removed)

2 cups peeled, sliced cucumber

$1/4$ cup coconut milk beverage

$1/4$ cup chia seeds

Combine all the ingredients in a
high-powered blender or food
processor and blend until smooth.

TOPPINGS

2 tablespoons toasted sliced almonds

2 tablespoons toasted unsweetened
flaked coconut

Sprigs of fresh mint leaves

Pour the smoothie into two small
bowls and sprinkle each with half
of the toppings and serve.

NUTRITION FACTS (GRAMS PER SERVING)
Calories 280, Fat 18, Protein 10, Carbs 28, Fiber 17, Net Carbs 11

Bananas contain potassium, which is an essential mineral that plays major roles in
blood pressure regulation, insulin resistance, and diabetes.

Creamy Avocado Berry Whip

This subtly sweet, creamy bowl is a delicious habit for increasing fiber, antioxidants, and healthy fats in your diet.

Serves 4

SMOOTHIE

$1/2$ avocado, pitted and peeled

$1/2$ banana, peeled

$1/2$ cup raspberries

$1/2$ cup coconut milk yogurt

$1/4$ cup hulled hemp seeds

Combine all the ingredients in a blender and blend until smooth.

TOPPINGS

$1/4$ cup blueberries

$1/4$ cup raspberries

2 tablespoons toasted unsweetened flaked coconut

2 tablespoons toasted hulled hemp seeds

Pour the smoothie into four small bowls and sprinkle each with one quarter of the toppings and serve.

NUTRITION FACTS (GRAMS PER SERVING)
Calories 200, Fat 13, Protein 6, Carbs 20 Fiber 4, NetCarbs 16

Raspberries contain raspberry ketone, a natural phenolic compound that has been found to promote lipolysis, which is the technical term for body fat breakdown and release (a.k.a. weight loss).

Dragon Dream

This bowl is a tropical dessert. Sweet dragon fruit balances the tartness of kiwi in this brilliant blend.

Serves 4

SMOOTHIE

1 kiwi, peeled
1/2 banana, peeled
1 cup chopped dragon fruit, rind removed
1/4 cup coconut milk beverage
1/4 cup chia seeds

Combine all the ingredients in a blender and blend until smooth.

TOPPINGS

1/4 cup peeled, sliced banana
1/4 cup peeled, sliced kiwi
1/4 cup toasted unsweetened flaked coconut

Pour the smoothie into four small bowls and sprinkle with one quarter of the toppings and serve.

NUTRITION FACTS (GRAMS PER SERVING)
Calories 270, Fat 13, Protein 7, Carbs 36, Fiber 11, NetCarbs 25

Red dragon fruit is a rich source of carotenoids that are found concentrated in the human eye. A diet rich in these nutrients provides protection against ocular disease.

Dragon Colada

This bowl is a healthy rendition of the classic drink. Chia seeds naturally thicken and provide anti-inflammatory omega-3 fatty acids.

Serves 4

SMOOTHIE

1/2 banana, peeled

1/2 cup chopped pineapple, rind removed

1/2 cup chopped dragon fruit

1/4 cup coconut milk beverage

1/4 cup chia seeds

1 teaspoon pure vanilla extract

Combine all the ingredients in a blender and blend until smooth.

TOPPINGS

1/4 cup peeled, sliced banana

2 tablespoons toasted unsweetened flaked coconut

Pour the smoothie into four small bowls and add one quarter of the toppings and serve.

NUTRITION FACTS (GRAMS PER SERVING)
Calories 180, Fat 8, Protein 5, Carbs 25, Fiber 8, NetCarbs 17

Chia seeds have the ability to reduce blood pressure in both treated and untreated hypertensive individuals.

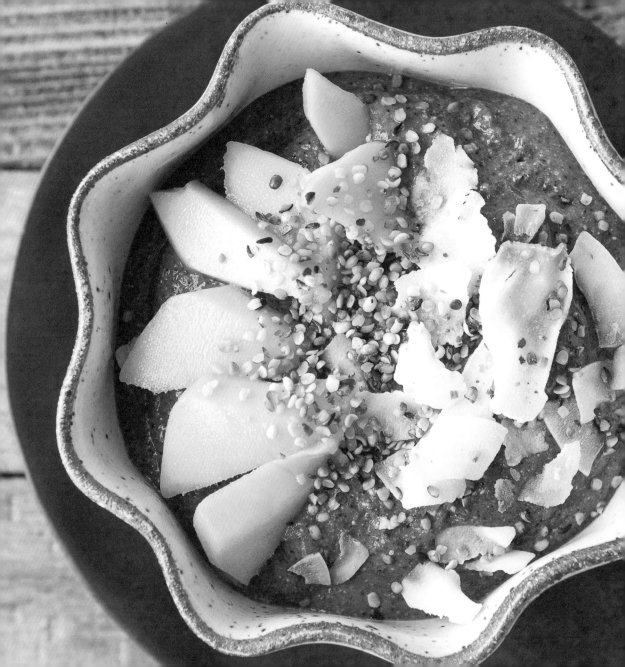

Mango Pineapple Lassi

Creamy and tangy from coconut milk yogurt, this bowl has both prebiotics and probiotics with wild blueberries that add potent antioxidants.

Serves 2

SMOOTHIE

1 cup chopped pineapple, rind removed

1 cup wild blueberries

1/2 cup pitted and peeled mango

1/2 cup coconut milk yogurt

1 teaspoon probiotic powder

Combine all the ingredients in a blender and blend until smooth.

TOPPINGS

1/2 cup pitted, peeled, and chopped mango

2 tablespoons toasted unsweetened flaked coconut

2 tablespoons toasted hulled hemp seeds

Pour the smoothie into two small bowls and sprinkle each with half of the toppings and serve.

NUTRITION FACTS (GRAMS PER SERVING)
Calories 280, Fat 10, Protein 6, Carbs 41, Fiber 6, Net Carbs 35

Mangoes are rich in prebiotic fiber and probiotics that support probiotic growth. *Bifidobacterium bifidum, Bifidobacterium lactose, Lactobacillus gasseri, Lactobacillus plantarum,* and *Lactobacillus rhamnosus* powders support weight loss.

Mexican Cocoa

This spiced chocolate blend has creamy avocado
and cocoa powder for powerful antioxidant effects.

Serves 2

SMOOTHIE

1 banana, peeled
$^1/_2$ avocado, pitted and peeled
$^1/_2$ cup coconut milk beverage
$^1/_4$ cup chia seeds
2 tablespoons unsweetened cocoa powder
1 tablespoon ground cinnamon
1 tablespoon pure vanilla extract
Pinch of cayenne pepper
Pinch of salt

Combine all the ingredients in
a blender and blend until smooth.

TOPPINGS

2 tablespoons sliced almonds
2 tablespoons hulled hemp seeds
2 tablespoons chopped dried cherries
2 tablespoons cocoa nibs

Pour the smoothie into two small
bowls and sprinkle each with half
of the toppings and serve.

NUTRITION FACTS (GRAMS PER SERVING)
Calories 320, Fat 18, Protein 11, Carbs 43, Fiber 21, Net Carbs 22

Cocoa flavonoids reduce insulin resistance. The polyphenols in cocoa have been shown
to restore beta cells and enhance insulin-releasing activity and glucose uptake, providing effective therapeutic support for both type 1 and type 2 diabetes.

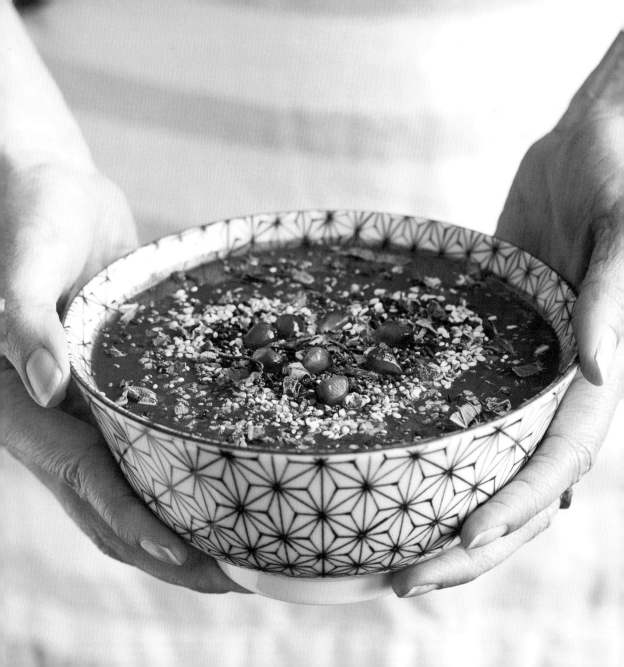

Personalized Therapeutic Smoothie Bowls

Personalize your bowls by adding foods that contain the nutrients you need to support your health conditions. These functional foods contain bioactive compounds proven to affect the following conditions.

Add $1/2$ to 2 cups of fruits or vegetables, 1 to 3 tablespoons of nuts and seeds, and 2 tablespoons of fresh or 1 teaspoon of dried herbs or spices to your daily bowl to reap the benefits of these healing foods.

THERAPEUTIC INGREDIENTS FOR SMOOTHIES

Anxiety

AVOCADO

BANANA AND ITS PEEL

BLACK PEPPER

CHIA SEEDS

COCOA POWDER

HULLED HEMP SEEDS

PROBIOTICS

PROTEIN POWDER

PUMPKIN SEEDS

TURMERIC

VANILLA

Arthritis

AVOCADO

BERRIES

BLACK PEPPER

CHIA SEEDS

CITRUS AND ITS PEEL

HULLED HEMP SEEDS

KALE

PROTEIN POWDER

SPEARMINT

SPINACH

TURMERIC

Back Pain

BANANA AND ITS PEEL

BASIL

BERRIES

BLACK PEPPER

CHIA SEEDS

NUTMEG

ROSEMARY

SESAME SEEDS

SPEARMINT

TURMERIC

WALNUTS

Bacterial and Fungal Infections

BANANA AND ITS PEEL

BASIL

BLACK PEPPER

CINNAMON

CITRUS AND ITS PEEL

CLOVES

GREEN TEA

MATCHA POWDER

OREGANO

PEPPERMINT

PROBIOTICS

PUMPKIN SEEDS

ROSEMARY

SPINACH

THYME

TURMERIC

Cancer

BERRIES

BLACK PEPPER

CILANTRO

CITRUS AND ITS PEEL

CLOVES

GINGER

GREEN TEA

KALE

MATCHA POWDER

NUTS

PAPAYA

POMEGRANATE

PROBIOTICS

RED GRAPES

SEEDS

SPINACH

STONE FRUIT

TURMERIC

WALNUTS

Cognitive Function

BANANA AND ITS PEEL

BERRIES

BLACK PEPPER

BLUEBERRIES

CASHEWS

CHERRIES

CITRUS AND ITS PEEL

KALE

MATCHA POWDER

PROBIOTICS

PROTEIN POWDER

SPINACH

STRAWBERRIES

TURMERIC

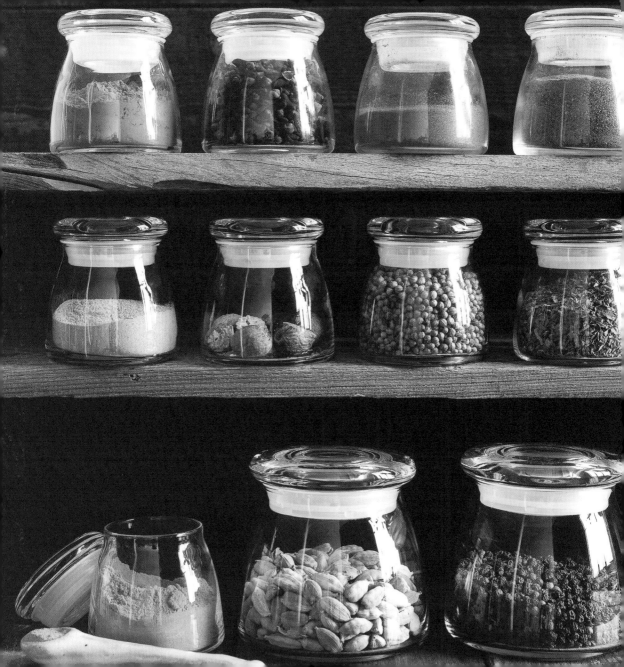

Dehydration

BANANA AND ITS PEEL

BERRIES

BLACK PEPPER

CITRUS AND ITS PEEL

KALE

POMEGRANATE

PROBIOTICS

SEEDS

SPINACH

TURMERIC

Dementia

BERRIES

BLACK PEPPER

BLUEBERRIES

CHERRIES

CHIA SEEDS

COFFEE

GREEN TEA

MATCHA POWDER

POMEGRANATE

PROBIOTICS

PROTEIN POWDER

SPINACH

STONE FRUIT

TURMERIC

Detox

AVOCADO

BANANA AND ITS PEEL

BASIL

CITRUS AND ITS PEEL

COCONUT
MILK YOGURT

KALE

MATCHA POWDER

MINT

OREGANO

PEPPERMINT

POMEGRANATE

PROBIOTICS

SPINACH

THYME

Diabetes

BANANA AND ITS PEEL

BLACK PEPPER

CARDAMOM

CASHEWS

CINNAMON

CITRUS AND ITS PEEL

COCOA NIBS

COCOA POWDER

GINGER

KALE

MATCHA POWDER

OREGANO

PROBIOTICS

PUMPKIN

PUMPKIN SEEDS

ROSEMARY

SEEDS

SPINACH

STONE FRUIT

THYME

TURMERIC

Digestion

HULLED HEMP SEEDS

PROBIOTICS

PROTEIN POWDER

PUMPKIN SEEDS

Dry Skin

AVOCADO

BERRIES

BLACK PEPPER

CHIA SEEDS

CILANTRO

PARSLEY

POMEGRANATE

PROBIOTICS

PROTEIN POWDER

PUMPKIN SEEDS

SEEDS

SPINACH

TURMERIC

Fatigue

BANANA AND ITS PEEL

BERRIES

BLACK PEPPER

CHIA SEEDS

CITRUS AND ITS PEEL

COCOA POWDER

COFFEE

COCONUT
MILK YOGURT

HULLED HEMP SEEDS

KALE

MATCHA POWDER

PROBIOTICS

PROTEIN POWDER

SPINACH

TURMERIC

Gastroesophageal Reflux Disease (GERD)

BANANA AND ITS PEEL

BERRIES

CASHEWS

COCONUT
MILK YOGURT

KALE

SPINACH

PARSLEY

PECANS

PROBIOTICS

PROTEIN POWDER

PUMPKIN SEEDS

Hair and Skin Health

BERRIES

BLACK PEPPER

BLUEBERRIES

CITRUS AND ITS PEEL

COCOA POWDER

NUTS

OREGANO

PEPPERMINT

POMEGRANATE

PROBIOTICS

SESAME SEEDS

THYME

TURMERIC

Headaches

BANANA AND ITS PEEL

BLACK PEPPER

COCOA POWDER

COFFEE

MATCHA POWDER

NUTS

SESAME SEEDS

SPINACH

TURMERIC

Heart Disease

AVOCADO	CHIA SEEDS	PAPAYA
BANANA AND ITS PEEL	COCOA POWDER	TURMERIC
BERRIES	GINGER	
BLACK PEPPER	NUTS	

High Blood Pressure

BANANA AND ITS PEEL
BERRIES
BLACK PEPPER
CHIA SEEDS
CLOVES
COCOA POWDER
GINGER
HAZELNUTS
MATCHA POWDER
NUTS
PECANS
SEEDS
TURMERIC

High Cholesterol

ALMONDS
AVOCADO
BERRIES
CARDAMOM
CHIA SEEDS
CINNAMON
GINGER
HULLED HEMP SEEDS
KALE
MATCHA POWDER
NUTS
PROBIOTICS
PROTEIN POWDER
SAFFRON
STRAWBERRIES

Hypoglycemia

APPLES
BERRIES
BLACK PEPPER
CHIA SEEDS
CINNAMON
CITRUS AND ITS PEEL
COCOA POWDER
COFFEE
GINGER
GRAPEFRUIT
HULLED HEMP SEEDS
KALE
MATCHA POWDER
NUTS
PROBIOTICS
PROTEIN POWDER
PUMPKIN SEEDS
ROMAINE LETTUCE
SEEDS
STRAWBERRIES
TURMERIC

Insomnia

BANANA AND ITS PEEL

BASIL

CHERRIES

CHIA SEEDS

COCONUT
MILK YOGURT

KIWI

LETTUCE

PROBIOTICS

PROTEIN POWDER

STRAWBERRIES

WALNUTS

Joint Pain

AVOCADO

BASIL

BERRIES

BLACK PEPPER

CHIA SEEDS

CITRUS AND ITS PEEL

CLOVES

GINGER

HULLED HEMP SEEDS

MINT

NUTS

PROTEIN POWDER

RED PEPPER

ROSEMARY

SPEARMINT

TURMERIC

VANILLA BEANS

WALNUTS

Muscle Cramps

AVOCADO

BANANA AND ITS PEEL

CASHEWS

CILANTRO

KALE

NUTS

PARSLEY

PROTEIN POWDER

SEEDS

SESAME SEEDS

SPINACH

Memory Loss

BANANA AND ITS PEEL

BERRIES

BLUEBERRIES

CHERRIES

CHIA SEEDS

CITRUS AND ITS PEEL

KALE

MATCHA POWDER

PEACHES

POMEGRANATE

PROBIOTICS

ROSEMARY

SPINACH

Overweight

APPLES

BANANA AND ITS PEEL

BERRIES

BLACK PEPPER

BLUEBERRIES

CHIA SEEDS

COCOA POWDER

COCONUT

COFFEE

CRANBERRIES

GRAPEFRUIT

KALE

LETTUCE

MANGO

MATCHA POWDER

PARSLEY

PEACHES

PROBIOTICS

ROMAINE LETTUCE

SESAME SEEDS

STRAWBERRIES

TURMERIC

Underweight

ALMONDS

AVOCADO

CASHEWS

CHIA SEEDS

HULLED HEMP SEEDS

PROBIOTICS

PROTEIN POWDER

UTIs (Urinary Tract Infections)

BLACK PEPPER

CRANBERRIES

OREGANO

PEPPERMINT

POMEGRANATE

PROBIOTICS

PUMPKIN SEEDS

SPINACH

THYME

TURMERIC

Viral Infections

APPLE

BERRIES

KALE

MATCHA POWDER

PROBIOTICS

PROTEIN POWDER

PUMPKIN

PUMPKIN SEEDS

SESAME SEEDS

SPINACH

STRAWBERRIES

Vision Impairment

BERRIES

CARROT JUICE

CINNAMON

CITRUS AND ITS PEEL

CLOVES

KALE

PEACH

PROBIOTICS

PUMPKIN

ROMAINE LETTUCE

SPINACH

Wrinkles

ANTIOXIDANTS

AVOCADO

BERRIES

BLACK PEPPER

CHIA SEEDS

CITRUS AND ITS PEEL

COCOA NIBS

COCOA POWDER

HULLED HEMP SEEDS

POMEGRANATE

PROBIOTICS

PUMPKIN

STONE FRUIT

TURMERIC

Resources

MIGHTY NEST | MIGHTYNEST.COM

MightyNest is a website that provides advice about toxins and home products. You can order natural, organic, and nontoxic products all in one place. All of its products are free from known toxic ingredients, such as BPA, PVC, phthalates, lead, melamine, formaldehyde, flame-retardants, parabens, and more.

ENVIRONMENTAL WORKING GROUP | EWG.ORG

The Environmental Working Group is an excellent resource for learning more about toxins in our homes, beauty products, and food. EWG is the creator of the Dirty Dozen and the Clean Fifteen lists, which report the most heavily sprayed produce and the least sprayed. These lists help us choose produce that is clean and avoid produce that test high in pesticides.

Acknowledgments

My deepest gratitude to Kristen Green Wiewora, Frances Soo Ping Chow, Amanda Richmond, Linda Konner, Olivia Brent, Sophie Elan, Patrick Jennings, Mimi Molotsky, McKenzie Johnson, Tara Booth, Linda Landkammer, Andrea Knutson, Cisca Schreefel, Iris Bass, Helen Gray, Anne Rierson, Cassidy Stockton, Susan Jardina, and my cultural attaché, Odette Jennings.

References

Agudelo-Ochoa, G. M., I. C. Pulgarín-Zapata, C. Velásquez-Rodriguez, M. Duque-Ramírez, M. Naranjo-Cano, M. M. Quintero-Ortiz, O. J. Lara-Guzmán, and K. Muñoz-Durango. "Coffee Consumption Increases the Antioxidant Capacity of Plasma and Has No Effect on the Lipid Profile or Vascular Function in Healthy Adults in a Randomized Controlled Trial." *Journal of Nutrition* (2016).

Akkasheh, G., Z. Kashani-Poor, M. Tajabadi-Ebrahimi, P. Jafari, H. Akbari, M. Taghizadeh, M. R. Memarzadeh, Z. Asemi, and A. Esmaillzadeh. "Clinical and Metabolic Response to Probiotic Administration in Patients with Major Depressive Disorder: A Randomized, Double-Blind, Placebo-Controlled Trial." *Nutrition* (2016).

Alasalvar, C., and B. W. Bolling. "Review of Nut Phytochemicals, Fat-Soluble Bioactives, Antioxidant Components and Health Effects." *British Journal of Nutrition* (2015).

Aleixandre, A., and M. Miguel. "Dietary Fiber and Blood Pressure Control." *Food Function* (2016).

Al-Karawi, D., D. A. Al Mamoori, and Y. Tayyar. "The Role of Curcumin Administration in Patients with Major Depressive Disorder: Mini Meta-analysis of Clinical Trials." *Phytotherapy Research* (2016).

Amir Aslani, B., and S. Ghobadi. "Studies on Oxidants and Antioxidants with a Brief Glance at Their Relevance to the Immune System." *Life Sciences* (2016).

Araújo Silva, V., J. Pereira da Sousa, H. de Luna Freire Pessôa, A. Fernanda Ramos de Freitas, H. Douglas Melo Coutinho, L. Beuttenmuller Nogueira Alves, and E. Oliveira Lima. "*Ocimum basilicum*: Antibacterial Activity and Association Study with Antibiotics Against Bacteria of Clinical Importance." *Pharmaceutical Biology* (2016).

Arun, K. B., F. Persia, P. S. Aswathy, J. Chandran, M. S. Sajeev, P. Jayamurthy, and P. Nisha. "Plantain Peel—A Potential Source of Antioxidant Dietary Fibre for Developing Functional Cookies." *Journal of Food Science and Technology* (2015).

Azimi, P., R. Ghiasvand, A. Feizi, M. Hariri, and B. Abbasi. "Effects of Cinnamon, Cardamom, Saffron, and Ginger Consumption on Markers of Glycemic Control, Lipid Profile, Oxidative Stress, and Inflammation in Type 2 Diabetes Patients." *Review of Diabetic Studies* (2014).

Bae, J., J. Kim, R. Choue, and H. Lim. "Fennel (*Foeniculum vulgare*) and Fenugreek (*Trigonella foenum-graecum*) Tea Drinking Suppresses Subjective Short-Term Appetite in Overweight Women." *Clinical Nutrition Research* (2015).

Barbagallo, C. M., A. B. Cefalù, D. Noto, and M. R. Averna. "Role of Nutraceuticals in Hypolipidemic Therapy." *Frontiers in Cardiovascular Medicine* (2015).

Benedec, D., D. Hanganu, I. Oniga, B. Tiperciuc, N. K. Olah, O. Raita, C. Bischin, R. Silaghi-Dumitrescu, and L. Vlase. "Assessment of Rosmarinic Acid Content in Six Lamiaceae Species Extracts and Their Antioxidant and Antimicrobial Potential." *Pakistan Journal of Pharmaceutical Sciences* (2015).

Benson, C., K. Mifflin, B. Kerr, S. J. Jesudasan, S. Dursun, and G. Baker. "Biogenic Amines and the Amino Acids GABA and Glutamate: Relationships with Pain and Depression." *Modern Trends in Pharmacopsychiatry* (2015).

Bernstein, P. S., B. Li, P. P. Vachali, A. Gorusupudi, R. Shyam, B. S. Henriksen, and J. M. Nolan. "Lutein, Zeaxanthin, and Meso-zeaxanthin: The Basic and Clinical Science Underlying Carotenoid-Based Nutritional Interventions Against Ocular Disease." *Progress in Retinal and Eye Research* (2016).

Bertoia, M. "Intake of Apples, Peppers and Other Foods High in Flavonoids Helps Prevent Weight Gain." *Nursing Standard* (2016).

Boyanapalli, S. S., and A. N. Tony Kong. "Curcumin, the King of Spices: Epigenetic Regulatory Mechanisms in the Prevention of Cancer, Neurological, and Inflammatory Diseases." *Current Pharmacology Reports* (2015).

Burns, A. M., M. A. Zitt, C. C. Rowe, B. Langkamp-Henken, V. Mai, C. Nieves Jr., M. Ukhanova, M. C. Christman, and W. J. Dahl. "Diet Quality Improves for Parents and Children When Almonds Are Incorporated into Their Daily Diet: A Randomized, Crossover Study." *Nutrition Research* (2016).

Castro-Vazquez, L., M. E. Alañón, V. Rodríguez-Robledo, M. S. Pérez-Coello, I. Hermosín-Gutierrez, M. C. Díaz-Maroto, J. Jordán, M. F. Galindo, and M. Arroyo-Jiménez Mdel. "Bioactive Flavonoids, Antioxidant Behaviour, and Cytoprotective Effects of Dried Grapefruit Peels (*Citrus paradisi Macf.*)." *Oxidative Medicine & Cellular Longevity* (2016).

Chaves, D. S., F. S. Frattani, M. Assafim, A. P. de Almeida, R. B. de Zingali, and S. S. Costa. "Phenolic Chemical Composition of *Petroselinum crispum* Extract and Its Effect on Haemostasis." *Natural Product Communications* (2011).

Choi, S. J., S. Y. Park, J. S. Park, S. K. Park, and M. Y. Jung. "Contents and Compositions of Policosanols in Green Tea (*Camellia sinensis*) Leaves." *Food Chemistry* (2016).

Chowdhury, A., J. Sarkar, T. Chakraborti, P. K. Pramanik, and S. Chakraborti. "Protective Role of Epigallocatechin-3-Gallate in Health and Disease: A Perspective." *Biomedicine & Pharmacotherapy* (2016).

Chuengsamarn, S., S. Rattanamongkolgul, B. Phonrat, R. Tungtrongchitr, and S. Jirawatnotai. "Reduction of Atherogenic Risk in Patients with Type 2 Diabetes by Curcuminoid Extract: A Randomized Controlled Trial." *Journal of Nutrition and Biochemistry* (2014).

Cicero, A. F., and A. Colletti. "Role of Phytochemicals in the Management of Metabolic Syndrome." *Phytomedicine* (2015).

Cipriani, F., A. Dondi, and G. Ricci. "Recent Advances in Epidemiology and Prevention of Atopic Eczema." *Pediatric Allergy and Immunology* (2014).

Connelly, A. E., A. J. Tucker, H. Tulk, M. Catapang, L. Chapman, N. Sheikh, S. Yurchenko, R. Fletcher, L. S. Kott, A. M. Duncan, and A. J. Wright. "High-Rosmarinic Acid Spearmint Tea in the Management of Knee Osteoarthritis Symptoms." *Journal of Medicinal Food* (2014).

Costa, A., E. S. Pegas Pereira, E. C. Assumpção, F. B. Calixto Dos Santos, F. S. Ota, M. de

Oliveira Pereira, M. C. Fidelis, R. Fávaro, S. S. Barros Langen, L. H. Favaro de Arruda, and E. N. Abildgaard. "Assessment of Clinical Effects and Safety of an Oral Supplement Based on Marine Protein, Vitamin C, Grape Seed Extract, Zinc, and Tomato Extract in the Improvement of Visible Signs of Skin Aging in Men." *Clinical Cosmetic Investigative Dermatology* (2015).

Crichton, G. E., M. F. Elias, and A. Alkerwi. "Chocolate Intake Is Associated with Better Cognitive Function: The Maine-Syracuse Longitudinal Study." *Appetite* (2016).

de Oliveira, M. R. "The Effects of Ellagic Acid upon Brain Cells: A Mechanistic View and Future Directions." *Neurochemical Research* (2016).

Dagli, N., R. Dagli, R. S. Mahmoud, and K. Baroudi. "Essential Oils, Their Therapeutic Properties, and Implication in Dentistry: A Review." *Journal of International Society of Preventive and Community Dentistry* (2015).

Del Turco, S., and G. Basta. "Can Dietary Polyphenols Prevent the Formation of Toxic Compounds from Maillard Reaction?" *Current Drug Metabolism* (2016).

Dhandayuthapani, S., H. Azad, and A. Rathinavelu. "Apoptosis Induction by *Ocimum sanctum* Extract in LNCaP Prostate Cancer Cells." *Journal of Medicinal Food* (2015).

Di Giuseppe, D., A. Crippa, N. Orsini, and A. Wolk. "Fish Consumption and Risk of Rheumatoid Arthritis: A Dose-Response Meta-analysis." *Arthritis Research & Therapy* (2014).

Dikalov, S. I., and A. E. Dikalova. "Contribution of Mitochondrial Oxidative Stress to Hypertension." *Current Opinion in Nephrology and Hypertension* (2016).

Dreher, M. L., and A. J. Davenport. "Hass Avocado Composition and Potential Health Effects." *Critical Review Food Science Nutrition* (2013).

Ekmekcioglu, C., I. Elmadfa, A. L. Meyer, and T. Moeslinger. "The Role of Dietary Potassium in Hypertension and Diabetes." *Journal of Physiology and Biochemistry* (2016).

El-Shabrawi, M. H., N. M. Kamal, M. A. Elhusseini, L. Hussein, E. A. Abdallah, Y. Z. Ali, A. A. Azab, M. A. Salama, M. Kassab, and M. Krawinkel. "Folic Acid Intake and Neural Tube

Defects: Two Egyptian Centers' Experience." *Medicine (Baltimore)* (2015).

Fraga, C. G., and P. Oteiza. "Flavanols and Vascular Health: Molecular Mechanisms to Build Evidence-Based Recommendations." *Free Radical Biology & Medicine* (2014).

Fulton, A. S., A. M. Hill, M. T. Williams, P. R. Howe, P. A. Frith, L. G. Wood, M. L. Garg, and A. M. Coates. "Feasibility of ω-3 Fatty Acid Supplementation as an Adjunct Therapy for People with Chronic Obstructive Pulmonary Disease: Study Protocol for a Randomized Controlled Trial." *Trials* (2013).

Galland, L. "The Gut Microbiome and the Brain." *Journal of Medicinal Food* (2014).

Gamboa-Gómez, C. I., N. E. Rocha-Guzmán, J. A. Gallegos-Infante, M. R. Moreno-Jiménez, B. D. Vázquez-Cabral, and R. F. González-Laredo. "Plants with Potential Use on Obesity and Its Complications." *Experimental and Clinical Sciences, International Online Journal* (2015).

Garrido, M., J. Espino, D. González-Gómez, M. Lozano, C. Barriga, S. D. Paredes, and A. B. Rodríguez. "The Consumption of a Jerte Valley Cherry Product in Humans Enhances Mood, and Increases 5-Hydroxyindoleacetic Acid but Reduces Cortisol Levels in Urine." *Experimental Gerontology* (2012).

Gharami, K., M. Das, and S. Das. "Essential Role of Docosahexaenoic Acid Towards Development of a Smarter Brain." *Neurochem International* (2015).

Grassi, D., G. Desideri, F. Mai, L. Martella, M. De Feo, D. Soddu, E. Fellini, M. Veneri, C. A. Stamerra, and C. Ferri. "Cocoa, Glucose Tolerance, and Insulin Signaling: Cardiometabolic Protection." *Journal of Agriculture and Food Chemistry* (2015).

Grise, D. E., H. M. McAllister, and J. Langland. "Improved Clinical Outcomes of Patients with Type 2 Diabetes Mellitus Utilizing Integrative Medicine: A Case Report." *Global Advances in Health & Medicine* (2015).

Habtemariam, S. "The Therapeutic Potential of Rosemary (*Rosmarinus officinalis*) Diterpenes for Alzheimer's Disease." *Evidence Based Complementary and Alternative Medicines* (2016).

Hayaloglu, A. A., and N. Demir. "Phenolic Compounds, Volatiles, and Sensory Characteristics of Twelve Sweet Cherry (*Prunus avium L.*) Cultivars Grown in Turkey." *Journal of Food Science* (2016).

Heng, M. C. "Signaling Pathways Targeted by Curcumin in Acute and Chronic Injury: Burns and Photo-Damaged Skin." *International Journal of Dermatology* (2013).

Herman, A., K. Tambor, A. Herman. "Linalool Affects the Antimicrobial Efficacy of Essential Oils." *Current Microbiology* (2016).

Huang, H., Z. C. Ma, Y. G. Wang, Q. Hong, H. L. Tan, C. R. Xiao, Q. D. Liang, X. L. Tang, and Y. Gao. "Ferulic Acid Alleviates Aβ25–35- and Lipopolysaccharide-Induced PC12 Cellular Damage: A Potential Role in Alzheimer's Disease by PDE Inhibition." *International Journal of Clinical Pharmacology & Therapeutics* (2015).

Janssens, P. L., R. Hursel, and M. S. Westerterp-Plantenga. "Nutraceuticals for Body-Weight Management: The Role of Green Tea Catechins." *Physiology & Behavior* (2016).

Ji, Y., Z. Wu, Z. Dai, K. Sun, J. Wang, and G. Wu. "Nutritional Epigenetics with a Focus on Amino Acids: Implications for the Development and Treatment of Metabolic Syndrome." *Journal of Nutrition and Biochemistry* (2016).

Kanazawa, K., and H. Sakakibara. "High Content of Dopamine, a Strong Antioxidant, in Cavendish Banana." *Journal of Agricultural and Food Chemistry* (2000).

Keel, S., C. Itsiopoulos, K. Koklanis, M. Vukicevic, F. Cameron, H. Gilbertson, and L. Brazionis. "Dietary Patterns and Retinal Vascular Calibre in Children and Adolescents with Type 1 Diabetes." *Acta Ophthalmologica* (2016).

Kelly, D., R. F. Coen, K. O. Akuffo, S. Beatty, J. Dennison, R. Moran, J. Stack, A. N. Howard, R. Mulcahy, and J. M. Nolan. "Cognitive Function and Its Relationship with Macular Pigment Optical Density and Serum Concentrations of Its Constituent Carotenoids." *Journal of Alzheimer's Disease* (2015).

Kloubert, V., and L. Rink. "Zinc as a Micronutrient and Its Preventive Role of Oxidative Damage in Cells." *Food Function* (2015).

Kobyliak, N., C. Conte, G. Cammarota, A. P. Haley, I. Styriak, L. Gaspar, J. Fusek, L. Rodrigo, and P. Kruzliak. "Probiotics in Prevention and Treatment of Obesity: A Critical View." *Nutrition & Metabolism (London)* (2016).

Kozłowska, M., A. E. Laudy, J. Przybył, M. Ziarno, and E. Majewska. "Chemical Composition and Antibacterial Activity of Some Medical Plants from Lamiaceae Family." *Acta Poloniae Pharmaceutica* (2015).

Kumar, N. "Neurologic Aspects of Cobalamin (B12) Deficiency." *Handbook of Clinical Neurology* (2014).

Kwak, J. Y., S. Park, J. K. Seok, K. H. Liu, and Y. C. Boo. "Ascorbyl Coumarates as Multifunctional Cosmeceutical Agents That Inhibit Melanogenesis and Enhance Collagen Synthesis." *Archives of Dermatology Research* (2015).

Lademann, J., T. Vergou, M. E. Darvin, A. Patzelt, M. C. Meinke, C. Voit, D. Papakostas, L. Zastrow, W. Sterry, and O. Doucet. "Systemic and Combined Application of Antioxidants on the Barrier Properties of the Human Skin." *Skin Pharmacology and Physiology* (2016).

Lambert, J. E., J. A. Parnell, J. Han, T. Sturzenegger, H. A. Paul, H. J. Vogel, and R. A. Reimer. "Evaluation of Yellow Pea Fibre Supplementation on Weight Loss and the Gut Microbiota: A Randomized Controlled Trial." *BMC Gastroenterology* (2014).

Lançon, A., R. Frazzi, and N. Latruffe. "Anti-oxidant, Anti-inflammatory and Anti-angiogenic Properties of Resveratrol in Ocular Diseases." *Molecules* (2016).

Laribi, B., K. Kouki, M. M'Hamdi, and T. Bettaieb. "Coriander (*Coriandrum sativum L.*) and Its Bioactive Constituents." *Fitoterapia* (2015).

Lee, J., J. Y. Cho, S. Y. Lee, K. W. Lee, J. Lee, and J. Y. Song. "Vanillin Protects Human Keratinocyte Stem Cells Against Ultraviolet B Irradiation." *Food Chemical Toxicology* (2014).

Lee, S. Y., Y. O. Jung, J. G. Ryu, H. J. Oh, H. J. Son, S. H. Lee, J. E. Kwon, E. K. Kim, M. K. Park, S. H. Park, H. Y. Kim, and M. L. Cho. "Epigallocatechin-3-Gallate Ameliorates Autoimmune Arthritis by Reciprocal Regulation of T Helper-17 Regulatory T Cells and Inhibition of Osteoclastogenesis by Inhibiting STAT3 Signaling." *Journal of Leukocyte Biology* (2016).

Lee, Y. Y., E. J. Lee, J. S. Park, S. E. Jang, D. H. Kim, and H. S. Kim. "Anti-inflammatory and Antioxidant Mechanism of Tangeretin in Activated Microglia." *Journal of Neuroimmune Pharmacology* (2016).

Li, F., X. W. Yang, K. W. Krausz, R. G. Nichols, W. Xu, A. D. Patterson, and F. J. Gonzalez. "Modulation of Colon Cancer by Nutmeg." *Journal of Proteome Research* (2015).

Loffredo, L., L. Perri, C. Nocella, and F. Violi. "Antioxidant and Antiplatelet Activity by Polyphenol-Rich Nutrients: Focus on Extra-Virgin Olive Oil and Cocoa." *British Journal of Clinical Pharmacology* (2016).

Mahattanatawee, K., J. A. Manthey, G. Luzio, S. T. Talcott, K. Goodner, and E. A. Baldwin. "Total Antioxidant Activity and Fiber Content of Select Florida-Grown Tropical Fruits." *Journal of Agricultural & Food Chemistry* (2006).

Martin, M. Á., L. Goya, and S. Ramos. "Anti-diabetic Actions of Cocoa Flavanols." *Molecular Nutrition & Food Research* (2016).

Mathur, R., and G. M. Barlow. "Obesity and the Microbiome." *Expert Review of Gastroenterology and Hepatology* (2015).

McCabe, D., and M. Colbeck. "The Effectiveness of Essential Fatty Acid, B Vitamin, Vitamin C, Magnesium and Zinc Supplementation for Managing Stress in Women: A Systematic Review Protocol." *JBI Database of Systematic Reviews & Implementation Reports* (2015).

McIver, D. J., A. M. Grizales, J. S. Brownstein, and A. B. Goldfine. "Risk of Type 2 Diabetes Is Lower in US Adults Taking Chromium-Containing Supplements." *Journal of Nutrition* (2015).

Morin, C., P. U. Blier, and S. Fortin. "Eicosapentaenoic Acid and Docosapentaenoic Acid Monoglycerides Are More Potent Than Docosahexaenoic Acid Monoglyceride to Resolve Inflammation in a Rheumatoid Arthritis Model." *Arthritis Research & Therapy* (2015).

Naz, R. K., M. L. Lough, and E. K. Barthelmess. "Curcumin: A Novel Non-steroidal Contraceptive with Antimicrobial Properties." *Front Biosci (Elite Edition)* (2016).

Oikeh, E. I., E. S. Omoregie, F. E. Oviasogie, and K. Oriakhi. "Phytochemical, Antimicrobial, and Antioxidant Activities of Different Citrus Juice Concentrates." *Food Science Nutrition* (2015).

Patterson, E., P. M. Ryan, J. F. Cryan, T. G. Dinan, R. P. Ross, G. F. Fitzgerald, and C. Stanton. "Gut Microbiota, Obesity and Diabetes." *Postgraduate Medical Journal* (2016).

Peddada, K. V., K. V. Peddada, S. K. Shukla, A. Mishra, and V. Verma. "Role of Curcumin in Common Musculoskeletal Disorders: A Review of Current Laboratory, Translational, and Clinical Data." *Orthopedic Surgery* (2015).

Petyaev, I. M. "Lycopene Deficiency in Aging and Cardiovascular Disease." *Oxidative Medicine and Cellular Longevity* (2016).

Prasad, A. S. "Impact of the Discovery of Human Zinc Deficiency on Health." *Journal of Trace Elements in Medicine & Biology* (2014).

Redman, K., T. Ruffman, P. Fitzgerald, and S. Skeaff. "Iodine Deficiency and the Brain: Effects and Mechanisms." *Critical Reviews in Food Science and Nutrition* (2015).

Remely, M., I. Tesar, B. Hippe, S. Gnauer, P. Rust, and A. G. Haslberger. "Gut Microbiota Composition Correlates with Changes in Body Fat Content Due to Weight Loss." *Beneficial Microbes* (2015).

Rodriguez, E. B., M. L. Vidallon, D. J. Mendoza, and C. T. Reyes. "Health-Promoting Bioactivities of Betalains from Red Dragon Fruit Peels (*Hylocereus polyrhizus* [Weber] Britton and Rose) as Affected Bycarbohydrate Encapsulation." *Journal of the Science of Food & Agriculture* (2016).

Ros, E. "Nuts and CVD." *British Journal of Nutrition* (2015).

Rubey, R. N. "Could Lysine Supplementation Prevent Alzheimer's Dementia? A Novel Hypothesis." *Journal of Neuropsychiatric Disease and Treatment* (2010).

Russell, S. J., K. Hughes, and M. A. Bellis. "Impact of Childhood Experience and Adult Well-Being on Eating Preferences and Behaviors." *BMJ Open* (2016).

Sahebkar, A., C. Gurban, A. Serban, F. Andrica, and M. C. Serban. "Effects of Supplementation with Pomegranate Juice on Plasma C-reactive Protein Concentrations: A Systematic

Review and Meta-analysis of Randomized Controlled Trials." *Phytomedicine* (2015).

Sampath, C., Y. Zhu, S. Sang, and M. Ahmedna. "Bioactive Compounds Isolated from Apple, Tea, and Ginger Protect Against Dicarbonyl Induced Stress in Cultured Human Retinal Epithelial Cells." *Phytomedicine* (2016).

Scott, S. P., and L. E. Murray-Kolb. "Iron Status Is Associated with Performance on Executive Functioning Tasks in Non-anemic Young Women." *Journal of Nutrition* (2016).

Scripsema, N. K., D. N. Hu, and R. B. Rosen. "Lutein, Zeaxanthin, and Meso-zeaxanthin in the Clinical Management of Eye Disease." *Journal of Ophthalmology* (2015).

Sevindik, H. G., U. Ozgen, A. Atila, H. Ozturk Er, C. Kazaz, and H. Duman. "Phytochemical Studies and Quantitative HPLC Analysis of Rosmarinic Acid and Luteolin 5-O-☐-D-Glucopyranoside on *Thymus praecox* subsp. *grossheimii* var. *Grossheimii*." *Chemical and Pharmaceutical Bulletin (Tokyo)* (2015).

Shahar, S., S. Shafurah, N. S. Hasan Shaari, R. Rajikan, N. F. Rajab, B. Golkhalkhali, and Z. M. Zainuddin. "Roles of Diet, Lifetime Physical Activity and Oxidative DNA Damage in the Occurrence of Prostate Cancer Among Men in Klang Valley, Malaysia." *Asian Pacific Journal of Cancer Prevention* (2011).

Shinozaki, K., M. Okuda, S. Sasaki, I. Kunitsugu, and M. Shigeta. "Dietary Fiber Consumption Decreases the Risks of Overweight and Hypercholesterolemia in Japanese Children." *Annals of Nutrition and Metabolism* (2015).

Skrovankova, S., D. Sumczynski, J. Mlcek, T. Jurikova, and J. Sochor. "Bioactive Compounds and Antioxidant Activity in Different Types of Berries." *International Journal of Molecular Sciences* (2015).

Song, H., Z. Zheng, J. Wu, J. Lai, Q. Chu, and X. Zheng. "White Pitaya (*Hylocereus undatus*) Juice Attenuates Insulin Resistance and Hepatic Steatosis in Diet-Induced Obese Mice." *PLOS One* (2016).

Souza, P. R., and L. V. Norling. "Implications for Eicosapentaenoic Acid– and Docosahexaenoic Acid–Derived Resolvins as Therapeutics for Arthritis." *European Journal of Pharmacology* (2015).

Speirs, K. E., J. T. Hayes, S. Musaad, A. VanBrackle, and M. Sigman-Grant; All 4 Kids Obesity Resiliency Research Team. "Is Family Sense of Coherence a Protective Factor Against the Obesogenic Environment?" *Appetite* (2016).

Srinivasan, K. "Antioxidant Potential of Spices and Their Active Constituents." *Critical Reviews in Food Science and Nutrition* (2014).

St-Onge, M. P., T. Salinardi, K. Herron-Rubin, and R. M. Black. "A Weight-Loss Diet Including Coffee-Derived Mannooligosaccharides Enhances Adipose Tissue Loss in Overweight Men but Not Women." *Obesity (Silver Spring)* (2012).

Tamma, S. M., B. Shorter, K. L. Toh, R. Moldwin, and B. Gordon. "Influence of Polyunsaturated Fatty Acids on Urologic Inflammation." *International Urology and Nephrology* (2015).

Tarasov, E. A., D. V. Blinov, U. V. Zimovina, and E. A. Sandakova. "Magnesium Deficiency and Stress: Issues of Their Relationship, Diagnostic Tests, and Approaches to Therapy." *Ter Arkh* (2015).

Toscano, L. T., C. S. da Silva, L. T. Toscano, A. E. de Almeida, C. Santos Ada, and A. S. Silva. "Chia Flour Supplementation Reduces Blood Pressure in Hypertensive Subjects." *Plant Foods for Human Nutrition* (2014).

Tran, D., J. P. Townley, T. M. Barnes, and K. A. Greive. "An Anti-aging Skin Care System Containing Alpha Hydroxy Acids and Vitamins Improves the Biomechanical Parameters of Facial Skin." *Journal of Clinical, Cosmetic and Investigational Dermatology* (2015).

Trüeb, R. M. "The Impact of Oxidative Stress on Hair." *International Journal of Cosmetic Science* (2015).

Utzschneider, K. M., M. Kratz, C. J. Damman, and M. Hullar. "Mechanisms Linking the Gut Microbiome and Glucose Metabolism." *Journal of Clinical Endocrinology Metabolism* (2016).

Vecchio, A. L., J. A. Dias, J. A. Berkley, C. Boey, M. B. Cohen, S. Cruchet, I. Liguoro, E. S. Lindo, B. Sandhu, P. Sherman, T. Shimizu, and A. Guarino. "Comparison of Recommendations in Clinical Practice Guidelines for Acute Gastroenteritis in Children." *Journal of Pediatric Gastroenterology and Nutrition* (2016).

Walecka-Kapica, E., G. Klupnska, J. Chojnacki, K. Tomaszewska-Warda, A. Błonska, and C. Chojnacki. "The Effect of Melatonin Supplementation on the Quality of Sleep and Weight Status in Postmenopausal Women." Przeglad *Menopauzalny* (2014).

Whigham, L. D., and A. H. Redelfs. "Optical Detection of Carotenoids in Living Tissue as a Measure of Fruit and Vegetable Intake." *IEEE Engineering in Medicine and Biology Society. Annual Conference Proceedings* (2015).

Wojtunik-Kulesza, K. A., A. Oniszczuk, T. Oniszczuk, and M. Waksmundzka-Hajnos. "The Influence of Common Free Radicals and Antioxidants on Development of Alzheimer's Disease." *Biomedicine & Pharmacotherapy* (2016).

Yan, X., J. Tang, C. Dos Santos Passos, A. Nurisso, C. A. Simões-Pires, M. Ji, H. Lou, and P. Fan. "Characterization of Lignanamides from Hemp (*Cannabis sativa L.*) Seed and Their Antioxidant and Acetylcholinesterase Inhibitory Activities." *Journal of Agricultural and Food Chemistry* (2015).

Yoon, H. S., J. R. Kim, G. Y. Park, J. E. Kim, D. H. Lee, K. W. Lee, and J. H. Chung. "Cocoa Flavanol Supplementation Influences Skin Conditions of Photo-Aged Women: A 24-Week Double-Blind, Randomized, Controlled Trial." *Journal of Nutrition* (2016).

Zeng, Y., J. Yang, J. Du, X. Pu, X. Yang, S. Yang, and T. Yang. "Strategies of Functional Foods Promote Sleep in Human Being." *Current Signal Transduction Therapy* (2014).

Zhao, Y., D. X. Tan, Q. Lei, H. Chen, L. Wang, Q. T. Li, Y. Gao, and J. Kong. "Melatonin and Its Potential Biological Functions in the Fruits of Sweet Cherry." *Journal of Pineal Research* (2013).

Zhang, C. R., E. Jayashre, P. S. Kumar, and M. G. Nair. "Antioxidant and Anti-inflammatory Compounds in Nutmeg (*Myristicafragrans*) Pericarp as Determined by In Vitro Assays." *Natural Product Communications* (2015).

INDEX

Note: Page references in *italics* indicate photographs.

U

V